Supporting Successful Interventions in Schools

The Guilford Practical Intervention in the Schools Series

Kenneth W. Merrell, Founding Editor
T. Chris Riley-Tillman, Series Editor

www.guilford.com/practical

This series presents the most reader-friendly resources available in key areas of evidence-based practice in school settings. Practitioners will find trustworthy guides on effective behavioral, mental health, and academic interventions, and assessment and measurement approaches. Covering all aspects of planning, implementing, and evaluating high-quality services for students, books in the series are carefully crafted for everyday utility. Features include ready-to-use reproducibles, lay-flat binding to facilitate photocopying, appealing visual elements, and an oversized format. Recent titles have Web pages where purchasers can download and print the reproducible materials.

Recent Volumes

Promoting Student Happiness: Positive Psychology Interventions in Schools
Shannon M. Suldo

Effective Math Interventions: A Guide to Improving Whole-Number Knowledge
Robin S. Codding, Robert J. Volpe, and Brian C. Poncy

Emotional and Behavioral Problems of Young Children, Second Edition:
Effective Interventions in the Preschool and Kindergarten Years
Melissa L. Holland, Jessica Malmberg, and Gretchen Gimpel Peacock

Group Interventions in Schools: A Guide for Practitioners
Jennifer P. Keperling, Wendy M. Reinke, Dana Marchese, and Nicholas Ialongo

Transforming Schools: A Problem-Solving Approach to School Change
Rachel Cohen Losoff and Kelly Broxterman

Evidence-Based Strategies for Effective Classroom Management
David M. Hulac and Amy M. Briesch

School-Based Observation: A Practical Guide to Assessing Student Behavior
Amy M. Briesch, Robert J. Volpe, and Randy G. Floyd

Helping Students Overcome Social Anxiety: Skills for Academic and Social Success (SASS)
Carrie Masia Warner, Daniela Colognori, and Chelsea Lynch

Executive Skills in Children and Adolescents, Third Edition:
A Practical Guide to Assessment and Intervention
Peg Dawson and Richard Guare

Effective Universal Instruction: An Action-Oriented Approach to Improving Tier 1
Kimberly Gibbons, Sarah Brown, and Bradley C. Niebling

Supporting Successful Interventions in Schools:
Tools to Plan, Evaluate, and Sustain Effective Implementation
Lisa M. Hagermoser Sanetti and Melissa A. Collier-Meek

High-Impact Assessment Reports for Children and Adolescents:
A Consumer-Responsive Approach
Robert Lichtenstein and Bruce Ecker

Conducting School-Based Functional Behavioral Assessments,
Third Edition: A Practitioner's Guide
Mark W. Steege, Jamie L. Pratt, Garry Wickerd, Richard Guare, and T. Steuart Watson

Supporting Successful Interventions in Schools

Tools to Plan, Evaluate, and Sustain Effective Implementation

LISA M. HAGERMOSER SANETTI
MELISSA A. COLLIER-MEEK

THE GUILFORD PRESS
New York   London

Copyright © 2019 The Guilford Press
A Division of Guilford Publications, Inc.
370 Seventh Avenue, Suite 1200, New York, NY 10001
www.guilford.com

Printed in the United States of America

This book is printed on acid-free paper.

Last digit is print number: 9 8 7 6 5 4 3 2 1

Library of Congress Cataloging-in-Publication Data

Names: Hagermoser Sanetti, Lisa M., author. | Collier-Meek, Melissa A., author.
Title: Supporting successful interventions in schools : tools to plan, evaluate, and sustain
    effective implementation / Lisa M. Hagermoser Sanetti, Melissa A. Collier-Meek.
Description: New York : The Guilford Press, 2019. | Series: The Guilford practical intervention
    in the schools series | Includes bibliographical references and index.
Identifiers: LCCN 2018050388 | ISBN 9781462537730 (paperback)
Subjects: LCSH: School mental health services. | School psychology. | Learning disabled
    children. | Emotional problems of children | Behavior disorders in children. | BISAC:
    PSYCHOLOGY / Psychotherapy / Child & Adolescent. | MEDICAL / Audiology & Speech
    Pathology. | EDUCATION / Special Education / General. | SOCIAL SCIENCE / Social Work.
Classification: LCC LB3430 .H34 2019 | DDC 371.7/13—dc23
LC record available at *https://lccn.loc.gov/2018050388*

To Daniela, Matthew, and Iris
And to the thousands of adults
who work tirelessly every day to implement interventions
to support the academic, behavioral, and social–emotional needs
of all youth so that they can reach their potential
and achieve their dreams

About the Authors

Lisa M. Hagermoser Sanetti, PhD, BCBA, is Associate Professor in the School Psychology Program at the Neag School of Education, University of Connecticut, where she is also a Research Scientist at the Center for Behavioral Education and Research. She is a recipient of the Lightner Witmer Award for early-career scholarship in school psychology from Division 16 of the American Psychological Association. Dr. Sanetti is a licensed psychologist and Board Certified Behavior Analyst. Her research interests include implementation science, school-based mental health, and educator wellness. She is the author of over 60 journal articles and book chapters, as well as an edited collection on intervention fidelity, and she has made over 100 professional presentations.

Melissa A. Collier-Meek, PhD, BCBA, is Assistant Professor in the School Psychology Program at the University of Massachusetts Boston. She is a licensed psychologist and Board Certified Behavior Analyst. Dr. Collier-Meek consults with teachers, teams, and families to support intervention implementation and build multi-tiered systems of support to promote student behavioral and academic outcomes. Her research interests include implementation science, intervention fidelity assessment, feasible promotion strategies, and consultation. She is the author of over 35 journal articles and book chapters and has made over 80 professional presentations.

Preface

> - Have you developed an intervention to promote learner outcomes, only to realize the "implementer" isn't *actually* implementing it at all?
> - Have you trained someone to implement an intervention, only to find out a week later that he or she altered the intervention to the point that it was barely recognizable?
> - Have you sat in team meetings reviewing data for a learner who isn't progressing and believed it was because members of the team weren't implementing the plan, but you didn't know what to do?
> - Have you developed home-based interventions and realized that the parents can implement the intervention well, but often don't?
>
> **If you answered yes to any of the above questions, this book is for you.**

This book is for those who support the effective implementation of interventions. School psychologists, special educators, curriculum specialists, behavior analysts, supervisors, consultants: in such roles you work with educators and parents in school-, home-, and community-based settings to implement interventions for youth. Accessible chapters provide feasible, time-efficient, research-based strategies for getting interventions implemented with the ultimate goal of improving student outcomes. Although this may seem like a fairly straightforward task, implementation—the set of activities of putting an intervention into place—is a rapidly growing multidisciplinary field that addresses activities at the policy, organizational, intervention, and implementer levels. As such, the purview of implementation is quite large, and "getting interventions implemented" can take on a variety of different meanings. Thus, an important first goal before beginning the book is to establish what the focus of this book is and what it is not, and to be specific about what we mean by "getting interventions implemented."

The focus of this book is on what you can do *now* to help the educators, parents, and other implementers with whom you work to competently and consistently implement practices to improve youth outcomes. We recognize that there are policy, systems, and organizational factors in place that facilitate the implementation of interventions. We discuss them briefly, so that you are aware of what they are, but we do not focus on how to affect those factors. Why? Because change at that level is slow. Very, very slow. And there are youth who can benefit from your intervention expertise *now*. So, although we recommend that you consider what systems-level change could facilitate your professional practice, you will not learn how to effect that change in this book. However, you will learn the basics of implementation, how to make data-based decisions that take implementation into account, and a variety of strategies to get interventions implemented—now. Reproducible worksheets, strategy guides, and fidelity assessment tools can enable you to start supporting implementation now, and case studies illustrate how to put all the pieces together and bring the content to life.

Contents

PART I

FUNDAMENTALS

CHAPTER 1

Introduction to Intervention Implementation

Ideas are easy. Implementation is hard.
—GUY KAWASAKI

Over the past 30 years, the number of research-based interventions available to address learners' academic, behavioral, and social–emotional needs, as well as the measures to evaluate their outcomes, has skyrocketed. For learners to benefit from research-based interventions, however, they have to actually experience them. That is, someone (typically a teacher, instructional aide, or parent) has to *implement* the intervention as planned across time. For decades, it was assumed that once given an intervention plan and maybe some minimal training, the adult responsible for the intervention would rapidly be able to implement the intervention consistently across time. This assumption was wrong and resulted in generations of learners not receiving appropriate interventions, as designed, and thus having poorer outcomes than were necessary. This situation is unacceptable and yet it has continued.

Implementation has received increased attention since the early 2000s because of the response-to-intervention (RTI) movement. Suddenly, learners' responsiveness to a universal research-based intervention would be monitored and those who did not "respond" would quickly receive more intensive, targeted research-based intervention. Common sense tells you that **learners cannot respond to an intervention they did not receive.** Despite this obvious truism, the vast majority of schools does not collect implementation data and therefore cannot be sure whether interventions are being implemented as planned. Results of a recent evaluation of RTI suggested that learners' improvements were not as expected. Why? The research-based interventions were not being implemented as planned (Fuchs &

Fuchs, 2017). Despite the promise of a responsive, data-driven intervention delivery system, another generation of learners had poorer outcomes than necessary because of assuming, rather than ensuring, implementation will occur.

It is time to admit that, when it comes to systematically and proactively measuring and supporting implementation of research-based interventions, we have dropped the ball as a field. We now know that we can and we must do our best to improve our practice. We can and we must actively measure implementation and apply the numerous effective strategies for preventing low levels of implementation as well as those for promoting higher levels of implementation. Doing so will enable this generation of learners to receive research-based interventions *as they are intended* so that these learners can reach their full potential.

The purpose of this book is to provide the knowledge and tools you need to efficiently and effectively support another individual's implementation of an intervention toward the goal of improving learner outcomes. By incorporating the strategies in this book, you will learn how to make your intervention efforts (e.g., meeting with the implementer, collecting data, designing interventions) much more likely to effect a positive difference for the learner. Also, you will learn how to provide implementation support in a manner that is prevention-oriented and responsive, so that it is as low-intensity and resource-efficient as possible. To get started, we provide an introduction to the field of implementation and what it entails, explains why it's important to support intervention fidelity, and then describes how the content of this book can be incorporated into your current practice.

Throughout the book, we use the term "intervention" broadly to include academic, behavioral, and social–emotional prevention and intervention practices, programs, curricula, and innovations across levels (i.e., primary, secondary, tertiary). Because we expect that consultants (i.e., school personnel, coaches, colleagues, supervisors, etc., who are working to support another adult responsible for actually implementing the intervention) will be reading this book, we use the pronoun "you" throughout. We use the term "implementer" to refer to the teacher, instructional aide, parent, intern, etc., who is responsible for the ongoing implementation of the intervention. In most cases, the implementer is a single individual; however, it may also be a group, such as schoolwide team, responsible for delivering an intervention. Last, we use the term "learner" to refer to the person or group that is receiving the intervention.

IMPLEMENTATION 101

This book is designed to be practical guide to supporting implementation within your professional practice. It is not designed to provide a comprehensive overview of the rapidly growing implementation literature. That said, having a general understanding of what implementation involves will help you in your practice. Here, we provide a brief overview of implementation by defining the essential terms and then focus on one component of implementation specifically—intervention fidelity—and explain why it's critical to support intervention implementation in your practice.

What Is Implementation?

At the most basic level, implementation is the "to" in science *to practice* (Fixsen, Blasé, Duda, Naoom, & Van Dyke, 2010). In your setting, implementation is the link between an identified intervention and the desired changes in learner outcomes. Although this process seems pretty straightforward, we know from decades of research across multiple fields that implementation is highly complex. There is a wide range of theories, models, and frameworks used to explain, predict, and describe implementation (Nilsen, 2015). Reviewing all of these is beyond the scope of this book; suffice it to say that we know implementation can require a wide range of activities and processes and can be influenced by a wide range of variables at multiple ecological levels. Before diving into a brief review of the basics, let's clarify some terms. There are a lot of them, and because most include the word *implementation*, they are easily confused. Therefore, we discuss them in the following material, provide definitions in Table 1.1, and illustrate the relationship among them in Figure 1.1.

The term **"implementation"** refers to the set of activities and processes involved in putting a defined intervention into place in the functioning of a particular context (e.g., school, grade, classroom, home, community setting) to change practice patterns (Fixsen, Naoom, Blasé, Friedman, & Wallace, 2005; Forman et al., 2013; McHugh & Barlow, 2010). Within the implementation process there are both intervention activities and implementation activities (Fixsen et al., 2005). **"Intervention activities"** include the actions taken to deliver an intervention to a recipient in the implementation context. For example, an intervention activity could include a teacher providing behavior-specific praise as part of a behavior support plan, or a math specialist reviewing division problems with a student as part of an individualized education program. **"Implementation activities"** refer to the

TABLE 1.1. Definitions of Implementation Terms

Terms	Definitions
Implementation	The set of activities and processes of putting an intervention of known dimension into place in the functioning of a particular context to change practice patterns.
Intervention activities	The delivery of an intervention to an individual in the implementation context.
Implementation activities	The actions taken within the organizational context and related systems to support complete and appropriate intervention delivery.
Intervention outcomes	Indicators of whether the delivered intervention is having the intended effect on the individual receiving it.
Implementation outcomes	The effects of deliberate actions taken to implement an intervention.
Intervention fidelity	A specific type of implementation outcome that refers to the correspondence between the intervention as delivered and the intervention as described.

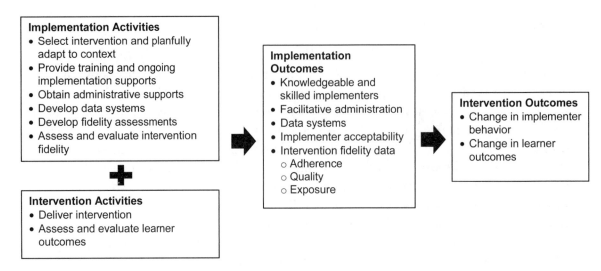

FIGURE 1.1. Relationship among and examples of implementation terms.

actions taken within the organizational context and related systems to support complete and appropriate intervention delivery. For example, an implementation activity could include a school psychologist meeting with a teacher to review the intervention plan.

"**Intervention outcomes**" are the effects of the intervention on the recipient. For example, intervention outcomes could include changes in scores on academic progress monitoring measures, frequency of occurrence of operationally defined behaviors, or changes in self-reports or teacher ratings of social–emotional well-being. "**Implementation outcomes**" are the effects of deliberate actions taken to implement an intervention; as such, they serve as prerequisites for intervention outcomes. For example, implementation outcomes include improved implementer knowledge and skill development, changes in perceived acceptability or feasibility, and levels of intervention fidelity.

"**Intervention fidelity**" (also commonly referred to as "treatment fidelity," "treatment integrity," "intervention integrity," or "procedural reliability") refers to the degree to which the intervention was implemented as prescribed or intended. As such, intervention fidelity is the aspect of implementation that is concerned with whether and how well the intervention actually got implemented. Estimates of the extent of intervention delivery, which you'll focus on evaluating and supporting in your practice, are considered measures of intervention fidelity. For example, the percentage of intervention steps implemented as planned daily or number of minutes for which an intervention is implemented would be considered measures of intervention fidelity. Intervention fidelity is often what individuals are referring to when they (incorrectly) use the term "implementation," and it is the primary focus of the rest of this book.

What Does Intervention Fidelity Entail?

Research over the past decade has shown that intervention fidelity is not a unidimensional construct focused on whether individual intervention components were or were not imple-

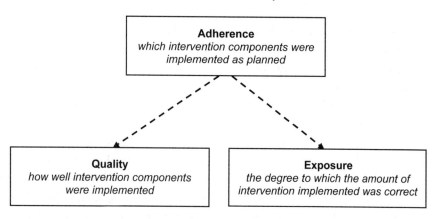

FIGURE 1.2. Empirically supported dimensions of intervention fidelity.

mented. We won't bore you with a detailed description of all the intervention fidelity frameworks (if you are interested, see Sanetti & Kratochwill, 2009, for a more extensive overview). Rather, we'll discuss the three dimensions that are fairly well agreed upon across these models and have been shown to improve data-based decision making (see Figure 1.2; Collier-Meek, Fallon, & DeFouw, 2018; Hirschstein, Edstrom, Frey, Snell, & MacKenzie, 2007; Sanetti & Fallon, 2011). The first is related to intervention content and is commonly referred to as **"adherence"**: that is, those intervention components that were implemented as planned. The second is related to **"quality"**: that is, how well intervention components were implemented. The third is related to quantity and is commonly referred to as **"exposure"**: that is, the amount of intervention implemented (e.g., number of sessions, duration of sessions; Power et al., 2005) as planned. Of these dimensions, adherence serves as a sort of gatekeeper in that without some level of adherence, you can't analyze quality or exposure.

Why Do We Have to Support Intervention Fidelity?

Now that you have the basic components of implementation, the next question you might have is "Why do I have to 'support' intervention fidelity?" For a lot of reasons, such as those outlined below.

Because We Know Implementers Need Support

It is important for intervention fidelity to be supported so that your assessment and intervention expertise can have a higher likelihood of resulting in improved learner outcomes. And, unfortunately, although we have a wealth of evidence-based interventions available to address the needs of youth, intervention fidelity in schools is relatively low (Ennett et al., 2003). Experience in practice as well as a wealth of research repeatedly demonstrates that, in the absence of implementation support, **most implementers struggle to deliver interventions as intended for more than 10 days** (Sanetti & Kratochwill, 2009). This has been found to be true across academic (Dufrene et al., 2012; Gilbertson, Willt, Singletary, Van-DerHeyden, 2007; Sundman-Wheat, Bradley-Klug, & Ogg, 2012) and behavioral (Collier-

Meek, Fallon, & DeFouw, 2017; Fallon, Collier-Meek, Sanetti, Feinberg, & Kratochwill, 2016; Jeffrey, McCurdy, Ewing, & Polis, 2009; Mouzakitus, Codding, Tryon, 2015; Sanetti, Collier-Meek, Long, Byron, & Kratochwill, 2015) interventions; at the individual (Fallon, Sanetti, Chafouleas, Faggella-Luby, & Welch, 2018; Mouzakitus et al., 2015; Sanetti et al., 2015; Gilbertson et al., 2007) and group (Collier-Meek et al., 2017; Dufrene et al., 2012; Jeffrey et al., 2009; Sanetti, Williamson, Long, & Kratochwill, 2018) levels; and in school (Gilbertson et al., 2007; Mouzakitus et al., 2015; Sanetti et al., 2015, 2018), home (Fallon et al., 2016; Sundman-Wheat et al., 2012), and community settings (Dufrene et al., 2012). Yet, **for decades upon decades we have assumed, but not supported, intervention fidelity.**

At first this reality may be a bit shocking, and after a while it may be a bit frustrating, but it is important to keep some perspective. **Intervention fidelity requires behavior change, and behavior change is hard. Really, really hard. For all of us.** If it weren't, we would all fulfill all of our New Year's resolutions. Every year. We know we certainly haven't fulfilled the vast majority of those resolutions. So, if behavior change is so hard, why do we think that when we present a new curriculum, group lesson, or individual intervention plan to implementers, that they will automatically change their behavior and implement it perfectly right away, with minimal training and little ongoing assistance? We are giving implementers a new set of skills, which may or may not be in their repertoire, to perform fluently and consistently, with minimal to no ongoing assistance or support, in addition to their current responsibilities. With this perspective, 0–10 days of adequate intervention fidelity is no longer surprising. **If you are not systematically and proactively supporting implementers, then you are actively not setting them up for success.**

Because Supporting Implementers Is Legally Required (in Some Situations)

If low levels of intervention fidelity aren't enough motivation, then let's consider your legal obligations to support implementation. Education legislation such as the Every Student Succeeds Act (2015) and the Individuals with Disabilities Education Act (2004) compel educators to use and evaluate evidence-based interventions to improve student outcomes. They don't say it is OK to just have knowledge of the evidence-based interventions; the law requires that such interventions *are actually used.* And "use" is intervention fidelity.

Further, the rapid adoption of multi-tiered systems of support (MTSS) as a delivery model for academic and behavioral interventions (e.g., RTI and schoolwide positive behavioral interventions and supports [PBIS]) has brought the importance of supporting intervention fidelity into focus (Kilgus, Collier-Meek, Johnson, & Jaffery, 2014). In MTSS models, high-quality curricula/interventions are delivered to all students, and regular assessment ensures that those students who are not making adequate progress receive more intensive interventions to meet their needs. Decisions about the intensity of student intervention are based on a *student's response* to a research-based intervention *implemented as planned* (National Center on Response to Intervention, 2010). Thus, in MTSS models in which implementation support is not provided, the odds are that interventions will not be delivered as intended, yet student outcomes will still be monitored, students will be found to be "not responsive" to the intervention (which they never really received), and a more intensive intervention will be (inappropriately) recommended.

When an MTSS model is used to determine eligibility for special education services, such as is allowable for specific learning disabilities in many states, then documentation of adequate intervention fidelity can be considered an essential due process protection (Noell & Gansle, 2006). As we know from the information above, implementing an intervention *as planned* typically requires support. So, to be able to document adequate intervention fidelity, you have to be capable of supporting implementers. If you aren't, the assessments, intervention development, progress monitoring, and data evaluation within MTSS are largely acts of futility.

Because Supporting Implementers Is Your Ethical Responsibility (Always)

Maybe you don't work in schools, so the bit about the legal responsibilities didn't convince you. But if you are delivering intervention services to youth in schools, homes, or communities, you likely have an ethics code by which you have said you will abide. Most ethics codes specify the need to provide effective intervention services; ensuring that an intervention is sufficiently implemented is necessary to be able to determine if it is effective. For example, the National Association of School Psychologists' (2010) *Principles for Professional Ethics* specifies that school psychologists provide effective services to children and youth and engage in effective decision making. Further, it states that before student disability labels are considered, the current practices and/or interventions should be fully evaluated. The American Counseling Association's (2014) *Code of Ethics* indicates that counselors should monitor the effectiveness of interventions, taking steps for improvement as appropriate (e.g., bolster intervention fidelity). The Behavior Analyst Certification Board's (2014) *Professional and Ethical Compliance Code* indicates that behavior analysts are expected to provide effective treatment to learners, which includes using evidence-based practice and monitoring the impact (and intervention fidelity) for individual learners. The Council for Exceptional Children's (2015) *Ethical Principles and Professional Practice Standards for Special Educators* indicates that special educators need to provide sufficient implementer training and use evidence-based practices that are monitored to evaluate effectiveness. If you are involved in delivering interventions to learners, you are likely ethically required to support implementers.

Because Supporting Implementers Works

For decades, we assumed intervention fidelity. When we assume that something is going well, then there is no need to assess it or figure out how to improve it. Since we took our collective heads out of the sand and recognized that we need to actively support implementers, our knowledge about intervention fidelity profiles and how to effectively support implementers has grown exponentially. A decade ago, there was one implementation support strategy being researched. Today there are dozens.

Implementation supports vary with regard to their focus (e.g., skill development, performance improvement) and intensity (e.g., amount of time and effort to deliver the support) because poor intervention fidelity doesn't always look the same or require the same level of support. For example, some individuals implement the whole intervention well but not often enough, whereas other individuals only implement certain intervention steps consistently and need support with adding additional intervention steps. Similarly, the strategies to support these implementers vary. Some individuals will be able to implement an intervention well after high-quality training alone, and will only need infrequent check-ins. Some individuals will have inadequate intervention fidelity after high-quality training, and will need a more intensive short-term support, whereas others require ongoing intensive support. The good thing is that whatever the pattern of intervention fidelity or type of strategy required, there is now a range of effective, theory-informed, and research-based implementation support strategies from which to choose (Noell et al., 2014). How to identify and deliver these implementation support strategies is the focus of this book. If you incorporate these strategies into your professional practice, you will be able to improve intervention fidelity and achieve improved learner outcomes.

SUPPORTING IMPLEMENTATION BY EMBEDDING THIS BOOK'S CONTENT INTO YOUR CURRENT PRACTICE

This book teaches you feasible, time-efficient, research-based, effective strategies to use during consultation or coaching to plan for intervention fidelity, prevent low levels of intervention fidelity, and promote intervention fidelity if or when levels decrease (see Figure 1.3). As such, your experience facilitating the data-driven identification and monitoring of evidence-based interventions will serve as the foundation for incorporating these implementation supports into your professional practice. We break down these prerequisite experiences in the following material, so you can be confident that you have the necessary knowledge and skill—or, if needed, how and where to reach out for additional training. Then we introduce the content and organization of the book so that you are ready to get started.

What Are the Skills and Foundational Knowledge?

Individuals who are responsible for providing implementation support are often also responsible for identifying and evaluating learner interventions. Intervention selection and evaluation typically occur as part of a problem-solving process (regardless of any specific consultation and coaching approach that you may use). To effectively integrate the content of this book into your practice, we expect that you can fluently engage in a problem-solving process that involves (1) working with an implementer to identify a learner concern to be addressed, (2) collecting baseline data, (3) confirming the presence of the concern and setting a goal, (4) identifying an intervention, and (5) assessing and evaluating learner progress. What we mean by each of these is briefly described next.

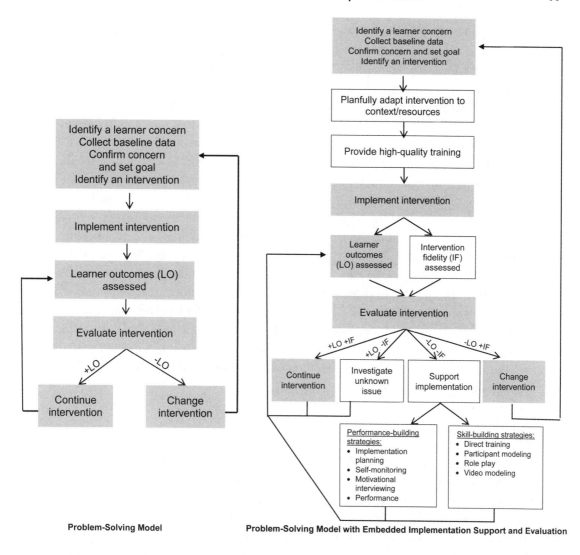

FIGURE 1.3. A typical problem-solving model and a problem-solving model with embedded implementation support and evaluation.

Working with Implementers to Identify a Learner Concern to Be Addressed

The implementation supports in this book are meant to be used in an indirect service delivery model, such as consultation and coaching, where you (as the consultant or coach) work with an implementer (e.g., teacher, parent) to support a learner. There are numerous consultation approaches, such as problem-solving consultation (also referred to as "behavioral consultation"; Bergan & Kratochwill, 1990), conjoint behavioral consultation (Sheridan & Kratochwill, 2007), and instructional consultation (Rosenfield, 1987). Although each consultation approach is unique, all involve efforts related to identifying the problem(s) to be addressed, analyzing the problem and developing an intervention, implementing an intervention, and evaluating the intervention. Coaching is similar to consultation in that it involves problem solving and identifying and evaluating interventions. It differs from consultation in that it has a strong emphasis on performance feedback and ongoing professional development (Schultz, Arora, & Mautone, 2015). Coaches are considered experts in the intervention and work with implementers in an ongoing basis to support implementation.

Regardless of your specific consultation or coaching approach, you should have experience collaborating and effectively communicating with implementers. To this end, it is essential to develop a positive and comfortable rapport. This relationship will serve as the foundation of your ongoing collaboration, so it is well worth the time to learn about the implementer and gain his or her buy-in for the consultation or coaching process. Once you have developed a rapport with the implementer, ask for his or her description of the concern to be addressed. Gather detailed information about what that concern looks like and the discrepancy between the current situation and what is expected. Throughout your communication with the implementer, be clear, positive, and avoid jargon. Regularly elicit, clarify, summarize, and validate the implementer's perspective. Work toward a definition of the concern that is observable (i.e., focused on characteristics that can be observed), measurable (i.e., written clearly to allow for consistent evaluation), and complete (i.e., clearly delineate boundaries of the concern; Cooper, Heron, & Heward, 2007). Such a definition will allow you and the implementer to identify specific goals for intervention outcomes and assess progress toward those goals across time.

Collecting Baseline Data

After a concern is operationalized, data should be collected. These data help you to ascertain whether the definition is appropriate and to document the occurrence of the concern prior to intervention. To determine how to collect baseline data, use your definition of the concern to inform your selection of a tool (e.g., test, observation tool, rating scale) that can quantify the construct, can be used repeatedly across time, and has adequate technical adequacy so that conclusions based on the resulting data are reliable and valid. To actually collect baseline data, you or another person should be able to apply the tool as it was meant to be used, which may involve facilitating some training.

Confirming the Presence of a Concern and Setting a Goal

After sufficient baseline data are collected, you will need to interpret the results. A discrepancy between the learner's outcomes and the expected outcomes suggests that there is a concern to be addressed. In this case, develop a specific, measureable, achievable, relevant, and time-bound (SMART) goal for the learner. This goal will serve as the foundation for evaluating the sufficiency of intervention fidelity (see discussion of data-based decision making in Chapter 3), so making sure that that it is data-driven, reasonable, and reflective of the implementer's concerns is critical. If the baseline data do not indicate a discrepancy between the learner's outcomes and the expected outcomes, we recommend that you discuss these results with the implementer and determine if the prior concern has greatly lessened or disappeared, or if adjustments to the problem definition or assessment approach may be necessary.

Identifying an Intervention

Based on the baseline data and learner goal, identify an evidence-based intervention. There are numerous criteria out there for determining what makes an intervention evidence-based versus bogus in pretty packaging. In general, however, an evidence-based intervention is one that has two or more studies that (1) randomly assign participants to conditions, (2) employ an appropriate design and high-quality methods, (3) result in statistically significant differences between the intervention group and the comparison group after intervention, and (4) are completed by different investigators (Kazdin & Weisz, 2010; Stoiber & DeSmet, 2010). There are numerous websites and books dedicated to identifying and listing evidence-based practices for different types of academic, behavioral, and social–emotional needs learners might have. Using an evidence-based intervention is ideal because before you even start to implement the intervention, you know it is likely to work. Of course, you still have to evaluate it to see if it works for the specific learner you are trying to help, but the evidence puts the odds in your favor.

Beyond evaluating the evidence base of an intervention, consideration of the context can also be important. Think about what is already present in the implementation context and whether you can to build on it. For example, if the implementer already incorporates a few components of a possible intervention as part of his or her daily routine, you may want to choose that intervention because it will build on current practices and may fit in the context better than other interventions. Taking a strengths-based approach to intervention identification (and to all aspects of the implementation support process) will facilitate a more positive interaction, allow the implementer to focus solely on new intervention components, and enable the implementer to experience implementation success quickly. If there are multiple evidence-based interventions of similar intensity that could be appropriate for the learner, involve the implementer in deciding which intervention is preferable. Providing help to the implementer when selecting the intervention has been shown to be related to higher levels of intervention fidelity (Dart, Cook, Collins, Gresham, & Chenier, 2012). Considering context and involving the implementer when identifying an intervention can go a long way to ensure that intervention activities are well received.

Assessing and Evaluating Learner Progress

Once an intervention is selected, data collection needs to continue to evaluate if the learner is making progress toward his or her goal. The same tool(s) used to collect baseline data should be applied to evaluate ongoing progress. Make sure that the intervention and data collection materials are easy to understand and use for the implementer. As intervention outcome data are continually collected, they can be used to identify whether the learner is or is not on track to meet his or her intervention goal within the identified timeline. Thus, make sure to check in regularly with the implementer throughout ongoing implementation.

Having this foundation in (1) working with the implementer to identify a learner concern, (2) collecting baseline data, (3) confirming the presence of the concern and setting a goal, (4) identifying an intervention, and (5) assessing and evaluating learner progress will make it possible to incorporate the content of this book into your professional practice. Specifically, we describe how to (1) promote intervention fidelity by planfully adapting interventions to fit the implementation context and providing high-quality training, (2) evaluate and make data-based decisions about intervention fidelity alongside learner outcomes, and (3) support intervention fidelity. If you do not feel comfortable with the concepts described here, reach out for additional training and supervision. Otherwise, let's discuss the book.

What's in the Rest of This Book?

Before diving into the implementation support strategies, we offer three foundational chapters. Chapter 2 provides an overview of how the practices related to intervention fidelity fit into the typical problem-solving process. Chapter 3 describes how to collect and graph intervention fidelity data so that you can recognize patterns in intervention implementation data. Chapter 4 discusses how to engage in data-based decision making, using implementation data and learner outcome data to determine an appropriate next step and, if needed, provide an appropriate form of implementation support. Here we present a multi-tiered framework for thinking about how to use these strategies to provide individuals with the type and level of implementation support they need—not more, not less.

From then on, the focus is solely on strategies to prevent low levels and promote high levels of intervention implementation. First, we describe implementation planning (Chapter 5) and direct training (Chapter 6), which are strategies that can be used to prevent or respond to low intervention fidelity. We recommend that both strategies be delivered prior to intervention implementation for all implementers; however, they can also be delivered in response to insufficient intervention fidelity. Next, we describe responsive strategies that can be delivered if and when there are low levels of intervention fidelity. Participant modeling and role play (Chapter 7), self-monitoring (Chapter 8), motivational interviewing (Chapter 9), and performance feedback (Chapter 10) are strategies designed to address skill and performance deficits that may be causing insufficient intervention fidelity. For each strategy, we briefly describe what you need to know about (1) what the strategy is, (2) research supporting the effectiveness of strategy, (3) how the strategy works, (4) who is most likely to benefit from the strategy, (5) how to prepare to deliver the strategy, (6) a detailed step-by-step description of how to deliver the strategy, and (7) how to follow up after you have delivered the strategy. Throughout all of it, we provide tables and figures to illustrate what we are talking about. Worksheets to facilitate documentation of data-based decision making, as well as reproducible protocols for each of the strategies, are also provided to support your professional practice. The book closes with case studies that illustrate how these implementation strategies and tools can be delivered to support implementers and improve learner outcomes.

By applying what you learn in this book to your practice, you will be equipped with (1) an understanding of the relationship between learner outcome data and intervention fidelity data, (2) a framework for thinking about differentiated implementation supports, and (3) a variety of strategies for addressing implementation issues. This knowledge will enable you to efficiently and differentially support intervention fidelity, thereby effectively improving recipient outcomes.

CHAPTER 2

Overview of Implementation Support and Evaluation within a Problem-Solving Model

In Chapter 1, we provided an overview of the broad field of implementation science and how intervention fidelity fits within it, why we need to support intervention fidelity, and what we expect you to already know. Now we are moving from *why* to *how*. In this chapter, we provide an overview of each of the steps of the problem-solving process with embedded implementation evaluation and supports. That is, we walk through the process you will go through as you work with an implementer to improve outcomes for a learner. Although we assume you are already competent in implementing the steps of the general problem-solving model, we describe them briefly in this chapter. There are numerous resources available that provide more in-depth coverage of these steps; we provide lists of such resources for you, should you want to deepen your problem-solving knowledge and skills. Specifically, Figure 2.1 (1) provides a description of various Internet-based resources available for you to immediately access information and (2) maps each of these resources to the stages of the problem-solving model. The remainder of the book is focused solely on providing the information and resources that you need to integrate the implementation-related steps into your practice.

THE PROBLEM-SOLVING PROCESS WITH EMBEDDED IMPLEMENTATION EVALUATION AND SUPPORTS

We assume that you already use a problem-solving process within your consultation or coaching work with implementers. This book provides additional tools and strategies you can use within your work to promote high-quality implementation. Figure 2.2 is a visual representation of the problem-solving model with embedded implementation evaluation

Resources	Identify learner concern	Collect baseline data	Confirm concern and set goal	Identify an intervention	Implement intervention	Assess learner outcomes	Evaluate intervention and make data-based decision
National Institute of Child Health and Human Development Review of research on how children learn to read and information on evidence-based methods for teaching reading. *www.nationalreadingpanel.org/Publications/summary.htm*				X	X		
Institute of Education Sciences Practice guides for research-based practices (WWC); videos and tools to apply research-based practices to schools. *http://ies.ed.gov/ncee/wwc* *http://dww.ed.gov*				X	X		
National Institute for Literacy Information on evidence-based literacy practices. *http://lincs.ed.gov*				X	X		
Office of English Language Acquisition Resources for meeting the instructional needs of English language learners. *www.ncela.gwu.edu*				X	X		
Intervention Central Information and resources for assessment and intervention related to individual, classwide, and schoolwide academic, behavioral, and social–emotional issues. *www.interventioncentral.org*	X	X	X	X	X	X	X
The IRIS Center Interactive training and evidence-based professional development resources for supporting students with disabilities. *http://iris.peabody.vanderbilt.edu*	X	X	X	X	X	X	X
Evidence-Based Intervention Network Descriptions and modeling videos of educational evidence-based frameworks. *http://ebi.missouri.edu*		X		X	X	X	
Best Evidence Encyclopedia Online resource for educators and researchers of scientific reviews of programs for children in grades K–12. *www.bestevidence.org*				X	X		
Council for Exceptional Children—Division for Learning Disabilities Online resource for educators of students with learning disabilities. *www.teachingld.org/ld_resources/default.htm*				X	X		

(continued)

FIGURE 2.1. Resources mapped to steps of the problem-solving process.

Resources	Identify learner concern	Collect baseline data	Confirm concern and set goal	Identify an intervention	Implement intervention	Assess learner outcomes	Evaluate intervention and make data-based decision
Florida Center for Reading Research Information on research-based literacy instruction and assessment practices for children in preschool through 12th grade. *www.fcrr.org*	X	X	X	X	X	X	X
Positive Behavioral Interventions and Supports—Office of Special Education Programs Technical Assistance Center Information on implementing positive behavioral interventions and supports, sponsored by the Department of Education. *www.pbis.org*	X	X	X	X	X	X	X
National Professional Development Center on Autism Information on evidence-based assessment and intervention practices for individuals with autism spectrum disorder. *http://autismpdc.fpg.unc.edu*				X	X		
Autism Internet Modules Online video training modules on how to implement evidence-based assessment and intervention practices for individuals with autism spectrum disorder. *www.autisminternetmodules.org/user_mod.php*	X	X	X	X	X	X	X
National Center on Intensive Intervention Resources (tools, charts, webinars) on evidence-based assessment and intervention practices for learners who need more intensive intervention to meet goals. *www.intensiveintervention.org*	X	X	X	X	X	X	X
National Implementation Research Network Resources on how to implement and sustain evidence-based practices in schools, districts, regions, and states. *http://nirn.fpg.unc.edu*				X	X		
Early Childhood Technical Assistance Center Resources on evidence-based practices for delivering high-quality early childhood education. *http://ectacenter.org/default.asp*	X	X		X	X	X	

FIGURE 2.1. *(continued)*

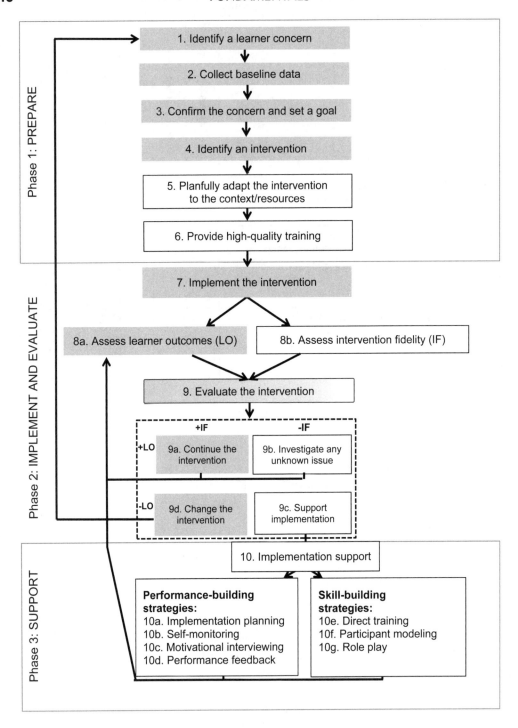

FIGURE 2.2. Problem-solving process with embedded implementation evaluation and supports. Shaded boxes represent typical steps of the problem-solving model. White boxes represent embedded implementation supports and evaluation. +LO, learner on track to meet goal; –LO, learner not on track to meet goal; +IF, sufficient intervention fidelity; –IF, insufficient intervention fidelity.

Problem-Solving Consultation Stages	Problem-Solving Process with Embedded Implementation Evaluation and Support	Instructional Coaching Stages
Problem Identification	1. Identify a learner concern 2. Collect baseline data 3. Confirm the concern and set a goal	Identify
Problem Analysis	4. Identify the intervention **5. Planfully adapt the intervention to the context/resources** **6. Provide high-quality training**	Learn
Plan Implementation	7. Implement the intervention 8a. Assess learner outcomes **8b. Assess intervention fidelity**	Improve
Plan Evaluation	9. Evaluate the intervention **10. Support implementation**	

FIGURE 2.3. Alignment of consultation and coaching stages with the problem-solving process and with embedded implementation evaluation and supports.

and supports. This figure depicts a stepwise process for beginning implementation with high levels of intervention fidelity, making data-based decisions about intervention effectiveness, and supporting intervention implementation when needed. **This process is aligned with typical consultation and coaching models** (see Figure 2.3; Kratochwill & Bergan, 1990; Knight et al., 2015) **and can be applied to any intervention** (e.g., reading, mathematics, social–emotional learning, behavioral supports) **at any scale** (e.g., individual learner, small group, schoolwide, agency). Although there certainly are differences depending on the type and scale of the intervention, the general problem-solving process should remain consistent.

As illustrated in Figure 2.2, this process includes 10 steps that occur across three phases; steps related to the general problem-solving model are shaded gray, and those related to implementation evaluation and supports are white. The first phase is focused on preparing

---

Quick Tip 2.1. Using the Implementation Tracking Log

The Implementation Tracking Log (see Appendix 2.1) can be used to keep track of your progress engaging in the problem-solving model with embedded evaluation support. This log can be copied and used by you for each implementer and learner whom you support. Keep the completed log to track all of the activities completed to identify an intervention, implement and evaluate it, and provide support. The Implementation Tracking Log includes all steps of the problem-solving model, with embedded evaluation support steps, as well as space for including action items, the person responsible, due date, and any notes. This log can be used use to indicate whatever individualized steps were completed (e.g., intervention fidelity schedule, decision made based on data review). That way, it will be a complete record of the problem-solving activities and ongoing support efforts.

A how-to guide for completing the Implementation Tracking Log is provided in Appendix 2.2. See Chapter 11 for case studies that illustrate the use of this worksheet in practice.

to implement an intervention and includes steps to facilitate your ability to begin implementation with high levels of intervention fidelity. It includes the typical problem-solving steps of identifying and analyzing the problem, as well as preparing the implementer for intervention implementation. The second phase is focused on implementation and evaluation and includes implementing the intervention, assessing learner outcomes and intervention fidelity, evaluating the intervention, and making a data-based decision. The third phase is focused on supporting implementation, when needed. It includes seven implementation support strategies you may use within your practice to increase intervention fidelity. Below we describe each step and provide a case example to illustrate the process.

Phase 1: Prepare

Step 1: Identify a Leaner Concern

Concerns about individual learners can come from a wide variety of sources. Teachers may be concerned about a learner who is consistently withdrawn from peers. Parents may contact the school because they notice that their learner can read words in some contexts, but seem to have never seen those words before in other contexts. A director of an after-school program may contact the school because a learner seems to have no clue how to do his or her homework. Benchmark data may result in the identification of learners as in need of additional intervention to meet an end-of-year learning goal. A paraprofessional or behavioral technician may raise a concern about a learner's lack of progress in his or her discrete trial instruction. Regardless of the source, it is essential to follow up on all learner concerns. Some may require intervention, some may not; but all indicate that there is a discrepancy between what is expected in a setting and what the learner is demonstrating.

To collect data to determine if the concern warrants intervention, it is essential to first define the concern. This is a typical starting point in the problem-solving model and involves having the individual who brought up the concern answer questions such as "What does [concern] look like?"; "When does it happen?"; and "How often does it occur?" A well-written definition will include three parts: (1) the conditions under which the problem is likely to occur; (2) a specific description of the problem; and (3) information about the frequency, intensity, duration, or other aspects of the concern that provide a context for estimating the extent to which the concern is discrepant from the expected outcomes (see Figure 2.1 for additional resources on defining learner concerns; Kratochwill, Altschaefl, & Bice-Urbach, 2014; Kratochwill & Bergan, 1990).

Case Example

A third-grade student named Lucy was referred by her teacher, Ms. Rosenberg, to the school psychologist, Mr. Hansen, because Lucy was regularly not following directions. After a conversation with Ms. Rosenberg about the noncompliance, the school psychologist learned that when Lucy is presented with a difficult (i.e., reading comprehension activities), nonpreferred task (e.g., reading aloud, putting math problems on the board)

Quick Tip 2.2. Using the Stranger Test

A useful method for determining whether a concern has been adequately defined is to apply the "stranger test." That is, if a stranger read the definition of the concern, then observed or interacted with the learner, would the stranger be able to reliably determine when the concern occurs and when it does not? If so, your definition meets the stranger test! If not, the definition needs further specification.

or a new task, Lucy is more likely to refuse to comply with the teacher's directions. Lucy's noncompliance typically involves putting her head on her desk and refusing to engage in the assigned task. Ms. Rosenberg reported that most students in the class are compliant with all tasks, and may only need a few reminders to stay on-task; Lucy, on the other hand, is noncompliant in most activities and it can take up to 5 minutes to get her reengaged.

Step 2: Collect Baseline Data

With the learner concern well defined, you can begin collecting baseline data. Depending on the concern, sufficient data may already be available. For example, a teacher may have data on a learner's reading skills that could be useful in understanding the extent of reading problems reported at home. In many cases, however, baseline data need to be collected using additional measurement tools. When collecting data, it is important to consider not only the learner, but also other factors that may be influencing the learner's outcomes. For example, regarding the reading concern, you may want to collect information about the quality and dosage of reading instruction, available reading materials at home and school, and the environment in the classroom and home during reading. Often baseline data include multiple types of data from multiple sources. These data should be carefully summarized and, in alignment with the definition of the concern, evaluated to determine if the concern about the learner suggests a need for intervention. Further, you will want to collect some baseline data using a measurement tool that also can be used for progress monitoring during intervention implementation (see Figure 2.1 for additional resources on collecting baseline data).

Case Example

To get a better understanding of the frequency of Lucy's noncompliance, Mr. Hansen (1) observed Lucy in the classroom three times during tasks Ms. Rosenberg reported were likely to result in noncompliance, and (2) gave Ms. Rosenberg a form on which to tally the number of instances of noncompliance each day for a week. Results of the three 20-minute observations indicated that (1) Lucy was noncompliant, on average, 2.3 times (range 1–4) across observations and (2) it took Ms. Rosenberg an average of 6 minutes (range 3–10) to reengage Lucy in the task. Ms. Rosenberg's data indicated that Lucy was noncompliant an average of 6.6 times (range 4–9) per day.

Step 3: Confirm the Concern and Set a Goal

With the baseline data summarized, determine whether a discrepancy between the learner's outcomes and the expected outcomes suggests that there is a concern to be addressed. If there is not a discrepancy, talk with the individual(s) who brought up the concern initially, discuss the baseline data, and determine the most appropriate next steps (e.g., adjustment of definition of concern, additional baseline data collection, collection of data in different setting, delay problem solving as student appears to be making sufficient progress). If there is a discrepancy, collaborate with the implementer and other relevant stakeholders (e.g., parents) to develop a SMART goal for the learner. You will use this goal when you evaluate intervention fidelity; that is, you will use it to answer the question of whether the intervention is being implemented sufficiently to facilitate the learner's progress toward this goal. So, take your time developing a goal that is data-driven, reasonable, and aligned with the identified learner concern (see Figure 2.1 for additional resources on setting goals).

Case Example

It was evident from review of the baseline data that there was a discrepancy between Lucy's frequency of noncompliance and that of her peers. Mr. Hansen and Ms. Rosenberg collaboratively developed the following goal for Lucy: When given a difficult, non-preferred, or new task, Lucy will engage in no more than an average of two instances of noncompliance per day by the end of the second marking term, as measured by frequency count collected by Ms. Rosenberg for 5 school days.

Step 4: Identify an Intervention

If the baseline data suggest that an intervention is needed, the next step is to identify appropriate evidence-based interventions or practices. As noted in Chapter 1, there are numerous websites and books dedicated to identifying and listing evidence-based practices for different types of needs learners might have (see Figure 2.1). Review the available interventions and select one that is aligned with the learner concern and seems reasonably feasible to implement in the relevant setting.

Case Example

Ms. Rosenberg indicated that she already differentiates all activities for her students, and will continue to do so to ensure that academic tasks are at Lucy's instructional level. Mr. Hansen and Ms. Rosenberg agreed to implement a behavioral intervention that included (1) setting the specific behavioral expectation ("Follow my teacher's directions the first time I'm asked"), (2) teaching Lucy what that behavior looks like through role plays based on typical classroom scenarios, and (3) implementing a differential reinforcement intervention. For the intervention, Ms. Rosenberg will create a list of potential reinforcers that are feasible and acceptable and have Lucy indicate which of those she is interested in earning; her choices will be noted on a reward menu. Per Ms. Rosenberg, there are nine natural breaks in the typical class routine. At the end of each of these breaks, Lucy will be able to put a sticker on a chart if she met the behavioral expectation since the prior break. Initially, if Lucy earns four stars, she will choose something from the reward menu. The number of stars to be earned will increase over time as she is successful.

Step 5: Planfully Adapt the Intervention to the Context/Resources

One of the realities of intervention implementation is that interventions that "fit" the context in which they are implemented are more likely to be implemented (Codding, Sanetti, & DiGennaro Reed, 2014). A related reality is that the clear majority of interventions get adapted in practice by implementers (Durlak & DuPre, 2008). Planful adaptations that take into consideration the theoretical and empirical basis of an intervention can facilitate use in practice; but adapting interventions haphazardly can result in several problems. First, haphazard adaptations can decrease the effectiveness of the intervention because typically, critical aspects of the intervention are changed or removed (Sanetti & Kratochwill, 2009). Second, often haphazard adaptations are not documented, so it is unclear what is being implemented consistently (Sanetti & Kratochwill, 2009). Thus, we recommend that you engage in implementation planning (Sanetti, Kratochwill, & Long, 2013; detailed in Chapter 5) with the implementer when you first introduce the intervention. Implementation planning allows you (as expert in the intervention) and the implementer (as expert in his or her setting or context) to sit together and make planful, documented adaptations to the intervention that maintain its critical aspects, yet better adapt the intervention to "fit" into the implementation context. In addition, implementation planning allows for early identification of the resources needed to implement the intervention. Further, implementation planning prompts the implementer to consider possible barriers to implementation and to develop strategies to address them proactively.

Case Example

With the intervention plan developed, Mr. Hansen led an implementation planning process with Ms. Rosenberg to ensure that the intervention would fit within the routines and context of her class. Ms. Rosenberg stated that she would (1) print the behavioral expectation on an index card and tape it to Lucy's desk to use as a prompt for her and (2) create a "unicorn" chart instead of a "star" chart for Lucy, given Lucy's interest in unicorns. Further, Ms. Rosenberg noted that she might need assistance from Mr. Hansen with maintaining rewards, depending on what Lucy chose. Finally, she and Mr. Hansen specified who would review the data and determine when Lucy's goal needed to be increased.

Step 6: Provide High-Quality Training

Although providing intervention training is embedded in most problem-solving consultation and coaching models, the realities of day-to-day practice often result in subpar training, if any, provided to implementers. We have pulled it out and made training its own action, because it is just that important. High-quality training that includes didactic instruction, modeling, practice, and feedback is prerequisite to sufficient intervention fidelity (Miles &

Wilder, 2009; Sterling-Turner, Watson, & Moore, 2002). We outline best practices in direct training in Chapter 6 and recommend that you deliver this training to all implementers, prior to intervention implementation, to provide them with the knowledge and skills needed to begin implementation with a high level of intervention fidelity. For some implementers, direct training will be sufficient to enable them to achieve satisfactory intervention fidelity (Sanetti & Collier-Meek, 2015). Others, however, will need additional implementation support to develop needed skills, deliver certain intervention skills consistently, and/or obtain/maintain motivation to implement the intervention (e.g., Mouzakitis et al., 2015; Noell, Witt, Gilbertson, Ranier, & Freeland, 1997; Romi & Teichman, 1998).

Case Example

Mr. Hansen knew that Ms. Rosenberg had implemented similar interventions previously, but he nevertheless provided training to Ms. Rosenberg because all plans are different and she did not feel confident responding to Lucy's noncompliance in the moment. They reviewed the rationale for the intervention and then took turns role-playing instructional situations in which Lucy might comply or not. First Ms. Rosenberg played Lucy and Mr. Hansen responded; then they traded roles. Overall, Ms. Rosenberg did a great job during the role plays, and Mr. Hansen provided constructive feedback about how to respond when Lucy is noncompliant or when she complies to the first request, but very slowly.

Phase 2: Implement and Evaluate

Step 7: Implement the Intervention

After choosing an evidence-based intervention, addressing intervention logistics and adaptations, and training the implementer, it is time for the implementer to deliver the intervention! (See Figure 2.1 for resources on intervention implementation beyond those provided in this book.)

Case Example

Ms. Rosenberg started implementing the intervention as soon as the reward menu and unicorn chart were created. Mr. Hansen checked in with Ms. Rosenberg weekly to address issues and answer questions.

Step 8a: Assess Learner Outcomes

Another cornerstone of problem-solving models is the ongoing monitoring of learner outcomes. Rather than waiting several months (or a whole year!) to measure the learner's progress, it is essential to measure progress formatively throughout intervention implementation. Ongoing progress monitoring with psychometrically sound measures provides half of the information needed to make a data-based decision about the effectiveness of the intervention. There are numerous commercially available, psychometrically sound instruments with which to measure learner progress across academic, behavioral, social–emotional domains; as mentioned above, you should have used one of these as part of your baseline data collection process (see Figure 2.1 for resources to identify an appropriate measure).

Case Example

Ms. Rosenberg collected frequency data on Lucy's noncompliance for 5 consecutive days each month. Further, Mr. Hansen observed Lucy's noncompliance once per week.

Step 8b: Assess Intervention Fidelity

The other half of the data needed to make a data-based decision about intervention effectiveness is intervention fidelity data. That is, to make decisions about intervention effectiveness, we must know if it was implemented as planned. Similar to learner progress, intervention fidelity should be measured formatively throughout intervention implementation (Sanetti, Fallon & Collier-Meek, 2011). Some interventions, particularly packaged interventions, include intervention fidelity measures. When psychometrically sound measures of intervention fidelity are available, use them! By doing so, you can be more confident in your interpretation of the data and subsequent decision making. When an intervention does not include a fidelity measure or is individualized for a learner, you will need to create your own measure (Sanetti et al., 2011). In Chapter 3, we provide guidance on how to develop an intervention fidelity tool to get you started in. That said, the science of intervention fidelity assessment is evolving rapidly, so it's a good idea to also regularly review best practice resources for up-to-date guidelines. Regardless of whether you are developing an intervention fidelity measure or using a previously validated measure, you will need to develop a plan for intervention fidelity data collection (e.g., how frequently, when, by whom). Depending on your data collection plan, you may need to train data collectors and you will need to set up a schedule for data review. We provide guidelines for all these logistical aspects in Chapter 3 as well.

Case Example

Mr. Hansen observed intervention fidelity three times per week for the first week, and weekly thereafter. He also created a self-report form on daily implementation practice that he asked Ms. Rosenberg to complete on randomly selected days.

Step 9: Evaluate the Intervention and Make a Data-Based Decision

With both intervention fidelity and learner outcome data, you can determine the extent to which the intervention was implemented and whether the learner is on track to meet their goal (Collier-Meek, Fallon, Sanetti, & Maggin, 2013). Because we assume that you are comfortable evaluating learner outcome data, we focus on how to evaluate intervention fidelity data and how to integrate it with learner outcome data. More specifically, in Chapter 4 we provide detailed guidance about how to graph, interpret, and summarize intervention fidelity data. Next, we discuss how to integrate learner outcome data and intervention fidelity data, the four possible resulting data profiles, and the next steps associated with each data profile. The four data profiles are described in detail in Chapter 4, and an overview is provided here. Data Profile A is evident when the learner is on track to meet his or her goal and intervention fidelity is sufficient. This data profile is the ideal scenario and suggests that the implementer should continue delivering the intervention, and you should continue to monitor learner outcomes and intervention fidelity. Data Profile B is evident when the learner is on track to meet his or her goal but intervention fidelity is insufficient. This data profile may initially seem confusing: How can a learner be making progress if the intervention is not being implemented well? Nevertheless, there are several reasons this profile might emerge, so we walk you through those and the associated next steps. Data Profile C is evident when the learner is not on track to meet his or her goal and intervention fidelity is insufficient. This data profile suggests the need for implementation support. There are seven implementation support strategies outlined in the next section of the book. In Chapters 5–10, we walk you through how you might use the available intervention fidelity data to decide which implementation support(s) to deliver, focusing on effectively supporting the implementer while using your time efficiently. Data profile D is evident when the learner is not on track to meet their goal but intervention fidelity is sufficient. Similar to Data Profile B, there are several reasons this profile might emerge, and we walk you through those and their associated next steps.

Case Example

After 2 weeks of implementation, Mr. Hansen and Ms. Rosenberg met to review Lucy's data and the intervention fidelity data. Lucy's noncompliance data showed a slight decreasing trend, but the slope of the line was insufficient for her to achieve her goal. Further, Ms. Rosenberg's intervention fidelity data were unacceptable. Although Mr. Hansen's observations suggested that Ms. Rosenberg was implementing the intervention sufficiently, Ms. Rosenberg's self-reported fidelity indicated that she consistently did not provide Lucy with the reward when it was earned. Overall, the data best fit Data Profile C.

Phase 3: Support

Step 10: Support Implementation

If the learner is not on track to meet his or her goal and the intervention is not being delivered sufficiently (i.e., Data Profile C), implementation support is needed. To identify the appropriate implementation support, we provide guidance regarding how to (1) consider implementation history, (2) review intervention fidelity data to evaluate whether the issue is best characterized as a skill or performance deficit, and (3) consider relevant strategies. Together, the information from these three steps will inform your selection of the implementation support strategy most appropriate for the implementer and the context. Each of the available implementation supports are briefly discussed in following material; the associated chapters include a description of (1) what the strategy is, (2) research supporting the effectiveness of strategy, (3) how the strategy works, (4) who is most likely to benefit from the strategy, (5) how to prepare to deliver the strategy, (6) a detailed step-by-step description of how to deliver the strategy, and (7) how to follow up after you have delivered the strategy.

STEP 10A: IMPLEMENTATION PLANNING

Implementation planning is one of two strategies that have been found to be effective when delivered as a preventive and a responsive form of support (e.g., Collier-Meek, Sanetti, & Boyle, 2016; Sanetti et al., 2015, 2018). As noted previously in Step 2, and described in detail in Chapter 5, the process of implementation planning allows you and the implementer to (1) make planful, documented adaptations to the intervention that maintain the critical aspects of the intervention; (2) improve the intervention's "fit" in the implementation context; (3) identify resources needed for implementation; and (4) identify and problem-solve anticipated barriers to implementation.

STEP 10B: SELF-MONITORING

When self-monitoring, the implementer attends to and rates his or her intervention fidelity (Petscher & Bailey, 2006; Plavnick, Ferreri, & Maupin, 2010; see Chapter 8). By doing so, the implementer is prompted to implement the intervention and thought to be reinforced by completing it with high fidelity (Cooper et al., 2007). Unlike other implementation supports in this book, the crux of this strategy is the implementer's engagement with ongoing self-monitoring, not a specific meeting. However, we do advise that you meet with the implementer to review the intervention, develop the self-monitoring form, practice completing it accurately, consider potential adaptations, and agree on a follow-up plan.

STEP 10C: MOTIVATIONAL INTERVIEWING

Motivational interviewing is a collaborative conversational approach to discussing behavior change that is intended to increase an individual's motivation for and commitment to change (Miller & Rollnick, 2013; see Chapter 9). Using this approach, you will guide a conversation about intervention fidelity and learner outcomes in which you positively respond to and evoke more implementer talk about being able to demonstrate sufficient intervention fidelity. Motivational interviewing is not focused on increasing an implementer's skill or fluency with intervention implementation. Rather, it is focused on increasing the implementer's motivation to implement consistently and comprehensively. There is a wide range of motivational interviewing techniques; we present a brief, simplified approach based on the elicit–provide–elicit technique, which has been used effectively to increase intervention implementation.

STEP 10D: PERFORMANCE FEEDBACK

Performance feedback is a form of implementation support that involves brief (5–15 minutes) meetings with an implementer to review and discuss intervention fidelity data (Noell et al., 1997, 2005; Solomon, Klein, & Politylo, 2012; see Chapter 10). During each meeting, you will praise the implementer for those intervention steps that are being implemented consistently, and highlight intervention steps that are being implemented poorly or not at all. You and the implementer may problem-solve why specific intervention steps are challenging to implement. Although each meeting is brief, performance feedback is designed to be delivered on an ongoing basis (e.g., weekly, or whenever intervention fidelity declines). The "critical components" of performance feedback target the goal of increasing the implementer's performance of intervention steps. That said, there are numerous ways to customize performance feedback, such as by including training, goal setting, self-management, or discussion of learner outcomes (Fallon, Collier-Meek, Maggin, Sanetti, & Johnson, 2015). We provide you with an overview of the critical components of performance feedback as well as the multiple ways you may customize it to best support the implementer.

STEP 10E: DIRECT TRAINING

Direct training is the second implementation support strategy that has been found to be effective when delivered as a preventive and a responsive form of support (Miles & Wilder, 2009; Sterling-Turner et al., 2002; see Chapter 6). In addition, direct training can be utilized during intervention implementation when intervention fidelity data or conversations with the implementer suggest a skill-based deficit. At this point, direct training can include a review of the entire intervention or can be focused on only those intervention steps the implementer isn't implementing consistently.

STEP 10F: PARTICIPANT MODELING

Participant modeling is an implementation support strategy that occurs over three sessions both in and outside of the implementation context (Collier-Meek, Sanetti, Levin, Kratochwill, & Boyle, 2018; Sanetti & Collier-Meek, 2015; Sanetti et al., 2018; see Chapter 7). First, you meet with the implementer and discuss intervention fidelity data and the intervention steps that are and are not being implemented sufficiently. Second, you model the accurate implementation of the intervention or specific intervention steps *in vivo* with the learner, with the implementer watching. Third, you provide an opportunity for the implementer to practice intervention implementation with you observing. Finally, you meet with the implementer to provide constructive feedback. Participant modeling is the only implementation support that includes *in vivo* practice. Although this can make it slightly more logistically challenging to deliver, it also makes it a highly efficient and effective way to support the implementer and address in-the-moment questions or concerns.

STEP 10G: ROLE PLAY

Role play is an implementation support strategy similar to participant modeling, in that it includes discussion of intervention fidelity data, modeling of intervention or intervention steps, implementer practice of the intervention or intervention steps, and provision of feedback to the implementer (Collier-Meek, Sanetti, et al., 2018; Joyce & Showers, 2002).

The primary difference is that role play occurs outside the implementation context, without the learner present, for modeling and implementer practice. Instead, the implementer will role-play as the learner while you model the intervention, and then you will role-play as the learner while the implementer practices. Because they are so similar, role play is presented in Chapter 7 along with participant modeling. In addition to describing the strategies, we provide guidance regarding how to decide if participant modeling or role play is the more appropriate strategy to support your implementer.

Case Example

Given that (1) Ms. Rosenberg's fidelity data indicated that she can implement the intervention sufficiently, but was regularly forgetting a few key steps (e.g., providing reward), and (2) Ms. Rosenberg consistently completed self-report forms related to implementation, Mr. Hansen decided to implement self-monitoring as a support to increase Ms. Rosenberg's implementation. Ms. Rosenberg agreed this would be a helpful prompt for her to remember all intervention steps and ensure that she implemented them as planned. Mr. Hansen and Ms. Rosenberg revised the draft self-monitoring form Mr. Hansen brought to their meeting and decided to conduct another data review in 2 weeks.

SUMMARY

In this chapter, we provided an illustration of how implementation evaluation and support can be embedded in a typical problem-solving model. We provided brief overviews of each component of the model and resources to gain more knowledge and skill related to problem solving. If, in your practice, you are not sure where to go next with an intervention case, we recommend that you reference Figure 2.2, the content in this chapter, and the Implementation Tracking Log (see Appendix 2.1 at the end of this chapter for a template of this log and Appendix 2.2 for a filled-in version) to reorient yourself so that you can move forward effectively and efficiently.

With a general idea of the steps for problem solving as well as implementation support and evaluation outlined, it is time to dive deeper into those steps unique to intervention fidelity. In the remaining nine chapters, we provide in-depth information about intervention fidelity assessment, data-based decision making, and the individual implementation supports. Each of these chapters is comprehensive and independent. That is, for example, if you want to implement a strategy, everything you will need (e.g., narrative description of each step, research support, strategy guide, associated intervention fidelity measure) is included in the chapter for that strategy. Let's dive in!

Implementation Tracking Log

Learner: _____

Consultant: _____

Implementers: _____

Intervention: _____

Use this worksheet to document the implementation process.

Date	Activity/Meeting	Action Steps	Person Responsible	Date Due	Notes
Phase 1: Prepare					
	1. Identify a learner concern				
	2. Collect baseline data				
	3. Confirm the concern and set a goal				
	4. Identify the intervention				
	5. Planfully adapt the intervention to the context/resources (i.e., provide implementation planning)				
	6. Provide high-quality training (i.e., direct training)				

(continued)

Implementation Tracking Log (page 2 of 2)

Date	Activity/Meeting	Action Steps	Person Responsible	Date Due	Notes
Phase 2: Implement and Evaluate					
	7. Implement the intervention				
	8a. Collect learner outcome data				
	8b. Collect intervention fidelity data				
	9. Evaluate the intervention and make data-based decisions (use Data-Based Decision-Making Worksheet)				
Phase 3: Support (as needed)					
	10. Support implementation				
	11. Evaluate the intervention				
	Repeat Steps 10 and 11 as needed.				

Guide for Completing the Implementation Tracking Log

Learner: Anthony, Gloria, Xander

Consultant: Mr. Wilson

Implementers: "Team A" seventh-grade teachers (Mr. Rodriguez, Ms. Blake, Ms. Garcia, Mr. Sullivan), CICO coordinator (Ms. Morales)

Intervention: CICO (all), math fluency intervention (Xander)

Use this worksheet to document the implementation process.

> 1. Record names and intervention.

> 2. List the start or meeting date for each activity.

> 3. List the activities and meetings to be completing during the problem-solving and implementation process (see Figure 2.1). These steps are initially standardized, but then individualize the activities and meetings based on the relevant data profiles.

> 4. Action steps are the specific next steps that need to be completed after each activity or meeting.

> 5. For each action step, identify the person responsible and the due date to make sure next that the steps are clear and to ensure follow-up.

> 6. Add notes, as needed, to keep track of the problem-solving and implementation process.

> 7. Keep it going! Add dates, activities, and action steps.

Date	Activity/Meeting	Action Steps	Person Responsible	Date Due	Notes
Phase 1: Prepare					
11/3	1. Identify learne...	...uct team meeting to operati... ...to collect baseline data	Consultant Consultant	11/5	
	...t baselin...	...ct behavior data (CICO form) ...ct CBM math data ...marize baseline data	"Team A" Ms. Blake Consulta...		
11/20	3. Confirm the c... a goal	...e if there is a concern to be addressed ...op SMART goals	Consulta... team Consultant		
11/22	4. Identify the int...	...n intervention materials ...op a draft of intervention fidelity materials	Consultant, CICO coordinator Consultant	12/1	
12/1	5. Planfully adapt the intervention to the context/ ...ovide ...anning)	• Share the implementation plan	Consultant	12/5	
	...ty training	• Train the implementers • Make sure the intervention materials are available to the implementers	Consultant, CICO coordinator Consultant, CICO coordinator	12/5	

From *Supporting Successful Interventions in Schools*, by Lisa M. Hagermoser Sanetti and Melissa A. Collier-Meek. Copyright © 2019 The Guilford Press. Permission to photocopy this material is granted to purchasers of the book for personal use or use with school personnel (see copyright page for details). Purchasers can download additional copies of this material (see the box at the end of the table of contents).

PART II

EVALUATION OF INTERVENTION FIDELITY AND LEARNER OUTCOMES

CHAPTER 3

Intervention Fidelity Data Collection

Once a learner concern is identified, it is critical to collect baseline data to identify patterns that can be used to target the intervention to the learner's specific needs and to facilitate the monitoring of the learner's response to the intervention across time (Cooper et al., 2007). Similarly, it is important to collect intervention fidelity data. In combination with learner outcome data, intervention fidelity data are used to target action steps (and implementation supports) specific to the implementer's needs and to facilitate the monitoring of the implementer's response to these supports across time (Sanetti & Collier-Meek, 2015). The process of evaluating intervention fidelity data on its own and in combination with learner outcome data to identify data-based next steps is the subject of Chapter 4. Before it is possible to engage in this decision making, however, you need to collect intervention fidelity data. Ideally those data would include measures of adherence (i.e., extent of intervention steps delivered), quality (i.e., how well intervention steps were implemented), and exposure (i.e., for how long the intervention was implemented; Collier-Meek, Fallon, & DeFouw, 2018; Hirschstein et al., 2007; Sanetti & Fallon, 2011). This chapter describes how to (1) document intervention delivery by providing data and (2) develop a plan to collect these data regularly. Throughout, you will consider the intensity of the intervention and related decisions (e.g., change of placement, special education eligibility) to decide what documentation methods and data collection plans you will utilize, with more intensive interventions and situations requiring more rigorous data collection. See the checklist in Figure 3.1 to review the steps involved in collecting intervention fidelity data.

DOCUMENTING INTERVENTION FIDELITY

To evaluate intervention fidelity, data must be collected systematically. Some interventions, particularly manualized ones, include intervention fidelity measures with the materials (e.g., Eames et al., 2007). Whenever psychometrically sound measures of intervention fidel-

✓	Intervention Fidelity Data Collection Steps
Document Intervention Fidelity	
	1. List the intervention steps
	2. Choose the assessment method
	3. Identify rating option(s)
	4. Pull the form together
Collect Intervention Fidelity Data	
	1. Train the data collector
	2. Determine the frequency of data collection
	3. Establish a schedule for regular data review

FIGURE 3.1. Intervention fidelity data collection steps.

ity are available, use them so that you can be more confident in your impression of intervention fidelity and subsequent decision making. When an intervention does not include these measures or when an intervention is individualized for a particular learner, you will need to create your own tool to document intervention fidelity (Sanetti et al., 2011). The science of how to develop an intervention fidelity tool is evolving quickly (Collier-Meek, Fallon, & Gould, 2018; DiGennaro Reed & Codding, 2014; Schulte, Easton, & Parker, 2009). We encourage readers to regularly review best-practice resources for up-to-date guidelines regarding intervention fidelity tools. Here we provide general guidelines and suggestions for a process of developing an intervention fidelity tool; these include (1) listing intervention steps, (2) choosing an assessment method, (3) identifying rating option(s), and (4) pulling together the form. As you go through this process, make sure to indicate any specific action steps, the person responsible, due date, and any notes on the Implementation Tracking Log (see Appendix 2.1, pp. 30–31).

Step 1: List the Intervention Steps

To measure how comprehensively and consistently an intervention is delivered, the specific intervention steps need to be listed and defined. This may be easier for some interventions than others. Review the intervention and list the specific steps necessary to implement it. Develop operational definitions for each intervention step that are observable (i.e., "What does this step look like?"), measurable (i.e., "Can I evaluate the occurrence of this step?"), and complete (i.e., "Does this account for all iterations of the intervention step?"; Cooper et al., 2007). Table 3.1 includes examples of intervention steps that are operationally defined. If you have already completed implementation planning (Chapter 5) and/or direct training (Chapter 6), you will already have a list of the intervention steps that you can use here. See Step 1 of the "Getting Ready for Implementation Planning" section of Chapter 5 (pp. 76–77) for additional guidance on how to divide an intervention into discrete steps.

TABLE 3.1. Examples of Intervention Steps

Intervention	Sample intervention steps
Schoolwide positive behavioral interventions and supports	• Tier 1 team meets at least monthly and has (1) regular meeting format/agenda, (2) minutes, (3) defined meeting roles, and (4) a current action plan.[a] • Expected academic and social behaviors are taught directly to all students in classrooms and across other campus settings/locations. • School has clear definitions for behaviors that interfere with academic and social success and a clear policy/procedure (e.g., flowchart) for addressing office-managed versus staff-managed problem behaviors.
Classroom management	• Praise statements—A teacher issues a verbal or nonverbal statement or gesture to provide feedback for a positive or appropriate behavior.[b] • Clear one- or two-step commands—A teacher delivers verbal instructions that request a specific behavior. These are clear and direct statements that provide explicit instructions to students. They are declarative statements (not questions) that clearly describe the desired behavior and include no more than two steps. • Academic response opportunities—A teacher creates opportunities for students to provide verbal academic responses (i.e., to answer or respond to lesson content questions, summarize content or key points, generate questions, brainstorm ideas, explain answer).
Direct instruction	• Preview lesson goals.[c] • Provide detailed explanation and instructions. • Show examples. • Provide frequent opportunities to respond. • Give regular feedback.
Cover, copy, compare math or spelling intervention	• Study sight word/math problem for 1 minute.[d] • Fold over paper to cover sight word/math problem. • Write sight word or complete math problem. • Compare written response to correct answer. • If incorrect, repeat cover, copy, compare sequence. • If correct, move to next sight word/math problem.
Individualized behavior support plan	• Post a visual reminder of the learner's behavioral expectations.[e] • Prompt the learner regarding the behavioral expectations prior to group-based work. • Provide behavior-specific praise when the learner demonstrates behavior according to the behavioral expectations. • Every 5 minutes, give the learner a smile or frown face on his or her behavior chart, paired with positive feedback. • At the end of the morning and afternoon, provide a reward if the learner has earned smiles for at least 50% of the intervals.
Discrete trial instruction	• Prompt for appropriate attending.[f] • Deliver academic prompt. • Wait 5 seconds for a response. • Deliver token and praise for correct responses. • Deliver least-to-most prompting for incorrect/no response.

[a]Items sampled with permission from SWPBIS Tiered Fidelity Inventory Version 2.1 (Algozzine et al., 2014).
[b]Effective classroom practices as defined in the Classroom Strategies Scale—Observer Form (Reddy, Fabiano, Dudek, & Hsu, 2013).
[c]See Wright (2013) for more information about direct instruction.
[d]See Skinner, McLaughlin, and Logan (1997) for more information about cover, copy, compare.
[e]See Sanetti and Collier-Meek (2014) for an evaluation of treatment integrity assessment of behavior support plans.
[f]See DiGennaro Reed, Reed, Baez, and Maguire (2011) for more information about discrete trial instruction.

As you define an intervention, consider the dimensions of intervention fidelity that are most relevant for each intervention step (Sanetti & Collier-Meek, 2014). In most cases, adherence, quality, and exposure are likely relevant (Sanetti & Fallon, 2011). Consider an intervention that requires the implementer to read a manualized script; a rating of adherence to the script and the quality of its delivery could be relevant. In addition, there could be an overall rating for exposure, or how long the intervention session lasted. For some intervention steps, only a specific dimension is applicable. Consider an intervention that requires the implementer to provide a token sheet to a learner weekly; for this intervention step, only adherence would likely be relevant.

To check if your list of intervention steps and definitions is sufficient, consider whether it would be possible to observe and measure each intervention step or to ask someone unfamiliar with the intervention if he or she clearly understood the intervention steps. If either of these ways of checking suggests that the listed steps do not sufficiently account for the entire intervention, revise your list and definitions. Examples of lists of complete intervention steps can be found in Chapter 11.

Step 2: Choose the Assessment Method

At this time, there are three assessment methods that can be used to document intervention fidelity: direct observation, permanent product review, and self-report. For *direct observation*, the delivery of the intervention plan is observed and either ratings are completed throughout the observation (e.g., records the frequency of behavior-specific praise; e.g., Collier-Meek, Johnson, & Farrell, 2018) or the extent to which specific intervention steps are rated are noted at the end of observation session (e.g., summary scores on a rating scale; Sanetti et al., 2015). Direct observation is the most versatile and direct assessment method; however, it can be time intensive (Sanetti & Collier-Meek, 2014). It is also possible that the implementer may act differently when an observer is present, although some research suggests that this is not the case (Codding, Livanis, Pace, & Vaca, 2008). Also, for some interventions—particularly those that are implemented for the whole day (e.g., behavior support plan)—it can be difficult to observe all of the intervention steps (Sanetti & Collier-Meek, 2014).

For *permanent product review*, materials used during the intervention can be reviewed after implementation to determine the degree to which the intervention steps were implemented (Cooper et al., 2007). For example, a learner's self-monitoring chart could be reviewed for estimates of intervention fidelity. Although not all interventions result in permanent products, when this assessment method is appropriate, such products can be unobtrusive and efficient (Noell et al., 1997, 2005).

For *self-report*, the implementer rates the extent of his or her intervention fidelity on a checklist or another form either throughout or after an intervention session (Ransford, Greenberg, Domitrovich, Small, & Jacobson, 2009). Self-report is a versatile method of intervention fidelity assessment that can be used across all types of interventions. It can serve as a prompt to remind implementers about all of the intervention steps. However, implementer self-reporting may not always be accurate, as human beings often (inadvertently!) overestimate their behavior (Noell et al., 2005).

When deciding among these options, consider the particular strengths and limitations of the assessment methods themselves, as well as their degree of "fit" with the situation at hand (Collier-Meek et al., 2013). That is, consider the intensity of the learner intervention and what decisions are likely to be made based on these data (e.g., increasing the intensity of the intervention, changing the learner's placement; Chafouleas, Riley-Tillman, & Sugai, 2007). **More intensive interventions or decisions call for a more direct intervention fidelity assessment method to be used.** That is, self-report alone is likely an inappropriate assessment method for interventions that are very resource-intensive or could result in a significant change in placement for the learner (Collier-Meek, et al., 2013). Other considerations include the match between an assessment method and the type of intervention, the relevant dimensions of intervention fidelity, the available resources, and the preferences of the implementer (Sanetti & Collier-Meek, 2014). For instance, the permanent product option may be appropriate for a low-intensity classwide intervention such as a token economy, when it is not feasible for you to observe regularly and the implementer does not mind dropping off intervention materials regularly.

In many cases, it may be possible and appropriate to use more than one assessment method to create an estimate of intervention fidelity (Sanetti & Collier-Meek, 2014). **This approach can balance the strengths and limitations of each assessment method.** You could choose to use both self-report and direct observation methods. For example, the implementer is asked to report implementation daily, and you will observe implementation on a monthly basis. This approach would allow for more frequent data collection (through self-report) as well as an accuracy check using a more direct method (through direct observation). In this situation, the direct observation data could also be used to give the implementer feedback about his or her self-ratings and help the implementer learn how to rate his or her own behavior more accurately. Consider multimethod assessment when the learner intervention or the related decisions are intensive. For instance, intervention fidelity assessment for an individualized function-based behavior support plan for a student with significant behavioral challenges might include implementer self-report, permanent product review of those steps that result in materials (e.g., reward chart), and biweekly direct observations. In another example, intervention fidelity assessment for a schoolwide Tier 1 behavior intervention might primarily involve quarterly self-reports from all implementers and additional direct observation for areas that have higher rates of challenging behaviors.

Step 3: Identify Rating Option(s)

Based on the intervention steps and assessment method(s) chosen, identify a way to rate the extent of intervention fidelity. You will provide ratings for each intervention step and each relevant intervention fidelity dimension. That is, if adherence and quality are applicable for a particular intervention step, then a separate rating is needed for each dimension of intervention fidelity. Possible rating options include a frequency count (i.e., tally when a step occurred; Cooper et al., 2007; Simonsen, MacSuga, Fallon, & Sugai, 2013), duration (i.e., list how long a step occurred for; Cooper et al., 2007; Sanetti & Fallon, 2011), time sampling (i.e., tally within an interval if a step occurred at any point [partial interval], for the entire interval [whole interval], or at the moment the interval changes [momentary time sampling];

Collier-Meek, Johnson & Farrell, 2018; Cooper et al., 2007), checklists (i.e., dichotomous rating of whether the step did or did not occur; Noell et al., 1997; Sanetti et al., 2011), Likert scales (i.e., a range of ratings from full implementation to no implementation; Sanetti et al., 2015), multiple-choice scales (i.e., a list of brief descriptions that correspond with different degrees of implementation), and fill in the blank (i.e., a space for a brief description in response to specific prompts/questions). The strengths and limitations of these options are listed in Table 3.2, and examples are illustrated in Table 3.3.

To decide among rating options, consider the intervention and context. Particular intervention steps and intervention fidelity dimensions may be best captured by specific ratings. For instance, a frequency count may capture adherence but not quality, whereas exposure may be best captured by duration. More direct ratings options (e.g., frequency counts, checklists, Likert scale) as opposed to more general methods (e.g., narrative response) may be more appropriate when interventions and related decisions are intensive (Chafouleas et al., 2007). Last, the resources available to facilitate data collection and rater or implementer preference may also influence the identified rating option. For example, an observer may be able to reliably collect frequency data, whereas an implementer completing a self-report form may not be able to do so, and a Likert scale rating may be more feasible and appropriate.

Step 4: Pull the Form Together

The last step in to preparing to document intervention fidelity is pulling the preceding steps together into an intervention fidelity tool. Based on the intervention steps, as well as the assessment method(s) and rating option(s) chosen, develop a data collection form to document the extent of intervention fidelity. List the intervention steps, identified above, on the form. Next, having identified appropriate rating options based on your assessment method, include a space for each rating option next to each intervention step. For example, each intervention step could have a corresponding yes/no or a Likert scale rating option. If evaluating for both adherence and quality, ensure that there is space for ranking both of these dimensions next to each step. In this case, you may have yes/no or a Likert scale rating option for adherence (i.e., to what extent did the implementer deliver each intervention step?) and quality (i.e., *how well* did the implementer deliver each intervention step?). You may rate exposure for individual intervention steps or for the whole intervention; depending on your decision, include space for this information next to each listed step or at the top or bottom of the form. Based on the intervention, assessment method(s), and rating option(s), this form may look very different. For examples, see Chapter 11.

COLLECTING INTERVENTION FIDELITY DATA

Once you have identified how you will document intervention fidelity, whether by a previously developed measure or a newly created tool, it needs to be used regularly. **To prepare, make sure the logistics of data collection are clear and feasible.** To plan for data collection, (1) train the individual(s) responsible for collecting the data, (2) determine the frequency of data collection, and (3) establish a schedule for regular data review.

TABLE 3.2. Strengths and Limitations of Rating Options

Type of rating	What is it?	Strengths	Limitations
Frequency count	Tally of when a step occurs	• Easy to develop, complete, and summarize	• Only useful for intervention steps for which the number of occurrences is the most important aspect of intervention fidelity • It may not be possible to accurately tally all intervention steps (e.g., if it occurs very frequently)
Duration	How long a step occurs for	• Easy to develop, complete, and summarize	• Only useful for intervention steps for which how long a step was implemented (i.e., exposure) is the most important aspect of intervention fidelity
Time sampling (partial interval, whole interval, or momentary time sampling)	Within intervals (e.g., 15 seconds, 1 minute), tally if the step occurs at any point, for the whole interval, or at the moment the interval changes	• Relevant for all dimensions of intervention fidelity • Relatively easy to develop, complete, and summarize	• May not account for the nuances of implementation or partial implementation
Checklist	Dichotomous rating of whether step did or did not occur	• Easy to develop, complete, and summarize	• May not account for the nuances of implementation or partial implementation
Likert scale	Range of ratings from full implementation to no implementation	• Relevant for all dimensions of intervention fidelity • Relatively easy to develop, complete, and summarize	• Decision rules need to be developed about what counts as "full" versus "partial" implementation
Multiple choice	List of brief descriptions that correspond with different degrees of implementation	• Relevant for all dimensions of intervention fidelity • Specific behavioral markers (e.g., schedule/goals reviewed, schedule or goals reviewed, no mention of schedule or goals) may increase consistency of ratings, as opposed to more general ratings (e.g., complete, partial, or not implemented)	• May be time-consuming to develop, as intervention steps may each require unique descriptions • Decision rules need to be developed about what counts as "full" versus "partial" implementation
Fill in the blank	Space for brief narrative in response to specific prompts/questions	• Relevant for all dimensions of intervention fidelity • Flexible format • Can account for nuances in implementation	• May be time-consuming to develop and complete • Responses will need to be converted to be analyzed; decision rules need to be developed about what counts as "full" implementation • Least direct rating method (may reflect rater's perspective rather than actual intervention fidelity)

TABLE 3.3. Examples of Rating Options

Type of rating	Adherence	Quality	Exposure
Frequency count	Tally of when the implementer provides behavior-specific praise.	Tally of when behavior-specific praise includes a reference to the behavioral expectations.	If the duration of the praise is of interest (e.g., implementer's praise is so long that it is interfering with instruction, or so brief that it is not being well received by the learner), you can record the duration, instead of tallying when the implementer provides behavior-specific praise. This will provide both a frequency count of the number of instances of behavior-specific praise as well as exposure data by instance.
Duration	Indicate the start and end time of the implementer actively supervising the hallway while students are changing classes.	Indicate for each minute of the passing period, whether the implementer was not simply standing in the hallway, but naturally moving around the space and providing behavior-specific praise to students.	Indicate the start and end time of the implementer actively supervising the hallway while students are changing classes.
Time sampling (partial interval, whole interval, or momentary time sampling)	Tally if any behavior-specific praise was provided within a 1-minute interval. Tally if implementer was actively supervising the classroom throughout a 15-second interval. Tally if the implementer was providing behavior-specific praise at the moment the 15-second interval changed.	Tally if behavior-specific praise that included a reference to behavioral expectations was provided within a 1-minute interval. Tally if behavior-specific praise involved positive, appropriate interactions throughout a 15-second interval. Tally if the implementer was providing behavior-specific praise that included a reference to behavioral expectations at the moment the 15-second interval changed.	Evaluate the percentage of intervals that included adherence or quality to get an estimate of exposure.
Checklist	When the student demonstrated safe behavior during circle time, was behavior-specific praise provided? • Yes • No	Was the behavior-specific praise delivered immediately with enthusiasm and reference to behavioral expectations? • Yes • No	Was the student present throughout circle time? • Yes • No

(continued)

TABLE 3.3. *(continued)*

Type of rating	Adherence	Quality	Exposure
Likert scale	When the student demonstrated safe behavior during circle time, was behavior-specific praise provided? • Implemented as planned • Implemented, but differently than planned • Not implemented	When provided, what was the quality of the behavior-specific praise? • Excellent • Good • Fair • Poor	The student was present throughout all of circle time. • Strongly agree • Agree • Neutral • Disagree • Strongly disagree
Multiple choice	When the student demonstrated safe behavior during circle time, was behavior-specific praise provided? • Following 100% of opportunities • Following half or more of opportunities • Following less than half of opportunities • Not provided following opportunities • No opportunity	When provided, what quality indicators of praise were present? • Behavior-specific • Contingent • Reference to behavioral expectations	When was the student present during circle time? • Throughout all of circle time • More than or equal to 50% of circle time • Less than 50% of circle time • Never attended circle time
Fill in the blank	Student demonstrated safe behavior on _____ occasions. Behavior-specific praise was provided on _____ occasions.	Provide an example of the praise provided: _____	Circle time lasted for _____ minutes. The student was present for _____ minutes.

Step 1: Train the Data Collector

To ensure that the intervention fidelity data are collected in an accurate and systematic manner, training is usually necessary (Cooper et al., 2007). That is, the data collector (e.g., implementer, assistant, consultant, coach) will need to learn about the assessment method generally and the intervention fidelity data collection form specifically (Sanetti et al., 2011). If the assessment method used does not require observation, it may still be helpful to train someone to collect, systematically review, and/or summarize the intervention fidelity data. Depending on the data collector, it might be useful to provide background information about intervention fidelity and the intervention itself. Preparing the data collector might include providing direct training (see Chapter 6), sharing a written guide to data collection, and practicing with you to ensure that both individuals are rating and summarizing intervention fidelity similarly. As you go through this process, make sure to indicate any specific action steps, the person responsible, due date, and any notes on the prepopulated or blank Implementation Tracking Log (Appendix 2.1, pp. 30–31).

Step 2: Determine the Frequency of Data Collection

To decide how frequently to collect intervention fidelity data, consider the situation and assessment method. When reviewing the situation, consider the intensity of the intervention as well as the type of decisions that will be made based on the intervention fidelity data (Chafouleas et al., 2007). For interventions that have greater intensity (e.g., learner is out of the classroom often, intervention requires substantial resources) assess intervention fidelity more frequently. Likewise, if high-stakes decisions will be made based on the data (e.g., intensity of learner intervention support, placement decisions), intervention fidelity should be assessed frequently. The method of assessment likely will impact the decision about how frequently to assess data as well (Sanetti & Collier-Meek, 2014). For instance, it is generally more feasible for an implementer to use a self-report method following each intervention session than for you to observe an intervention session daily.

Keep in mind that the data collection plan may change over time. For instance, it may be appropriate to collect intervention fidelity data frequently (e.g., daily) as the intervention is just getting started and then collect it less frequently (e.g., weekly) once levels of adherence stabilize. That said, **keep collecting intervention fidelity data throughout ongoing intervention delivery, as levels do change across time.** In many cases, implementers who start out delivering an intervention consistently can, over time, demonstrate lower, more variable intervention fidelity (e.g., Noell et al., 1997, Sanetti et al., 2015, 2011; Simonsen et al., 2013). Also, if intervention fidelity is low, it may be appropriate to collect data more frequently to evaluate the effectiveness of implementation support and provide more, if indicated (see Chapter 4).

Once the plan for how frequently intervention fidelity data will be collected is decided, develop a logistical plan to ensure follow-through. Record the dates on the Implementation Tracking Log (Appendix 2.1). For example, develop a calendar of intervention fidelity assessment dates with reminders and print copies of the intervention fidelity data forms. This advanced planning will ensure that intervention fidelity data are collected as planned.

Step 3: Establish a Schedule for Regular Data Review

To ensure the use of data-based decision making, intervention fidelity data must be reviewed regularly alongside learner outcome data (Collier-Meek et al., 2013). Although the specifics of this review are described in Chapter 4, for the purposes of developing an intervention fidelity data system, plan *when* intervention fidelity assessment data will be reviewed. As with the frequency of data collection, the frequency of the data review will depend on the intervention and situation (e.g., intensity of the decisions made based on the data). Once the frequency of data review is established, make sure that relevant stakeholders can be present for the meeting and that current intervention fidelity data and learner outcome data will be available and summarized to facilitate discussion. Record the dates for data review on the Implementation Tracking Log (Appendix 2.1).

SUMMARY

Before it is possible to engage in decision making about intervention effectiveness and learner outcomes, you need to collect intervention fidelity data. This chapter described how to document intervention delivery and develop a plan to collect these data regularly. Readers should use psychometrically sound intervention fidelity measures whenever available and regularly review best-practice resources for up-to-date guidelines on intervention fidelity tools. Based on currently available recommendations, guidelines for the process of developing an intervention fidelity tool include (1) listing intervention steps, (2) choosing an assessment method, (3) identifying rating option(s), and (4) preparing to summarize intervention fidelity data (Collier-Meek et al., 2013; Sanetti et al., 2011). Once an intervention fidelity tool is identified or developed, a plan for data collection that involves training the individual(s) responsible for collecting the data, determining the frequency of data collection, and establishing regular data review dates is needed (Collier-Meek et al., 2013; Sanetti et al., 2011). Review the checklist in Figure 3.1 to ensure that you are ready to collect intervention fidelity data. Once these data are collected, intervention fidelity can be evaluated separately and combined with learner outcome data to identify data-based next steps.

CHAPTER 4

Data-Based Decision Making
Considering Intervention Fidelity and Learner Outcome Data

Now that you have collected intervention fidelity data, it is time to evaluate these data and then evaluate them in relation to learner outcome data. Through this review you will identify the extent to which the intervention has been delivered with fidelity and how the intervention is related to the learner's subsequent response. Based on your prior experience, we expect that you are comfortable evaluating learner outcome data to identify if the learner is on track or not on track to meet his or her intervention goal (see Chapter 2 for more information and resources in this area). This chapter addresses how to evaluate intervention fidelity data in relation to learner outcome data to inform data-based decision making. First, we describe how to evaluate intervention fidelity data. Next, we explain how to integrate these data with information about the learner's outcomes to identify the relevant data profile. Last, we describe possible data profiles and outline specific action steps to guide your next steps.

EVALUATING INTERVENTION FIDELITY DATA

Although interventions need to be delivered consistently and comprehensively, there is no universal level of intervention fidelity that is necessary across all interventions (Gresham, 2014; Perepletchikova & Kazdin, 2005; Sanetti & Kratochwill, 2009). Some interventions need to be delivered with 100% adherence to efficiently and effectively impact learner outcomes (DiGennaro Reed, Reed, Baez, & Maguire, 2011; Wilder, Atwell, & Wine, 2006), whereas others can be delivered with 80% adherence (Sanetti et al., 2015) or even lower (e.g., 60% adherence; Durlak & DuPre, 2008). **So instead of looking for a specific level, you will summarize the intervention fidelity data and decide whether the specific intervention has been delivered to an extent that the learner could be reasonably expected to ben-**

efit from the intervention. To do so, we suggest that you summarize intervention fidelity data, graph these data, interpret these graphs, and then develop a statement to summarize current intervention fidelity. **Based on this interpretation of the intervention fidelity data, you will then decide whether there is (1) sufficient implementation or (2) insufficient implementation.** The steps for this process are described below.

Step 1: Summarize Intervention Fidelity

To facilitate evaluation and decision making, it is helpful to summarize the extent of intervention fidelity. There are two types of summary scores that are particularly useful in this regard—session intervention fidelity and intervention step fidelity—both of which can be evaluated for each intervention fidelity dimension assessed (see Table 4.1). *Session intervention fidelity* is calculated as the extent of intervention fidelity each time the intervention is supposed to be implemented (e.g., each intervention session, daily; Sanetti et al., 2011). For each dimension, session intervention fidelity can be assessed by answering specific questions. For example, for the dimension of adherence, you would ask "What percentage of intervention steps was implemented as planned during this session?" That is, session intervention fidelity for adherence is expressed as a percentage of steps delivered among all the applicable intervention steps. Depending on what rating method was used, you may be able to simply summarize the percentage of steps delivered as planned, or you may need to compare the data to a created standard (e.g., frequency of praise statements compared to expected number of praise statements). For quality, ask "What percentage of intervention steps was implemented with quality during this session?" That is, session intervention fidelity for quality is expressed as the percentage of steps delivered with quality among all intervention steps delivered. For exposure, ask "For how long did the implementer deliver the intervention?" Session intervention fidelity for exposure can be expressed directly (i.e., number of minutes) or as a percentage based on how long the intervention was supposed to be implemented (i.e., minutes implemented over minutes in the intervention protocol).

Intervention step fidelity refers to the extent to which specific intervention steps are implemented across sessions. Evaluating delivery of specific intervention steps facilitates

TABLE 4.1. Summary Scores across Intervention Fidelity Dimensions

Summary scores	Adherence	Quality	Exposure
Session intervention fidelity	What is the percentage of intervention steps implemented as planned during this session?	What is the percentage of intervention steps implemented with quality during this session?	For how long did the implementer deliver the intervention?
Intervention step fidelity	What is the extent to which a specific intervention step has been implemented over time?	To what extend has a specific intervention step been implemented with quality across time?	What is the average duration of exposure across time for a specific intervention step?

the review of patterns within intervention fidelity data. As with session intervention fidelity, intervention step fidelity can be assessed by answering specific questions. For adherence, "What is the extent to which a particular intervention step has been implemented across time?" Depending on what rating method is used, you may be able to summarize the percentage of times the particular intervention step was delivered as planned, or you may directly calculate the average number of times the intervention step occurred across sessions (e.g., mean frequency of praise statements for observations of equal lengths, mean rate of praise statements if observations are of different lengths, mean percentage of intervals that included behavior-specific praise). For quality, "To what extent has a particular intervention step been implemented with quality across time?" For exposure, "What is the average duration of exposure across time for a particular intervention step?" When calculating intervention step fidelity, you can summarize across all intervention sessions or consider specific intervention sessions (e.g., sessions in which a learner did really well, sessions before or after implementation support). Being able to review patterns for specific intervention steps allows for a targeted understanding of intervention fidelity. Calculating these types of summary scores will help you evaluate intervention fidelity data across time and will inform decisions to provide additional support to the implementers or to modify the intervention plan.

Case Example

Mr. Suen, a seventh-grade math teacher, is implementing the Good Behavior Game, a behavioral group contingency intervention that involves defining classroom expectations, grouping students into teams, tallying misbehaviors, and the providing a reward to the team that receives the fewest tallies (Barrish, Saunders, & Wolf, 1969). The school psychologist, Ms. Rodriguez, who is helping Mr. Suen deliver the game, has decided to summarize the intervention fidelity in three ways every time Mr. Suen's class plays the game. She will document the number of steps delivered as planned (session intervention fidelity for adherence), the number of steps implemented with quality (session intervention fidelity for quality), and the duration of the game (exposure). In addition, Ms. Rodriguez will review the intervention fidelity data across a week to see if specific intervention steps seem challenging (intervention step fidelity).

Step 2: Graph Data

Graphing can help you review patterns in data to facilitate accurate and nuanced interpretations (Burke, Howard, Peterson, Peterson, & Allen, 2012; Hood & Dorman, 2008; Sanetti, Luiselli, & Handler, 2007). Although there are many ways to graph data, here we provide specific suggestions for how to graph session intervention fidelity and intervention step fidelity, which can be applied across each dimension of intervention fidelity (i.e., adherence, quality, exposure; see Table 4.1). That is, we describe how session intervention fidelity data can be summarized in a line graph, and how intervention step intervention fidelity data can be summarized in a bar graph.

Because line graphs are most often used to summarize data across time, they are appropriate for illustrating the extent of intervention fidelity across varied sessions (see example

Quick Tip 4.1. Getting Help with Graphs

 Graphing data helps to illustrate patterns that can be identified through visual analysis (Kratochwill et al., 2010). To evaluate whether intervention fidelity is sufficient, we suggest that you regularly graph session intervention fidelity and intervention step fidelity. If you do not have experience graphing, the following resources might provide a helpful introduction.

WEBSITES

Intervention Central—ChartDog Graph Maker
www.interventioncentral.org/teacher-resources/graph-maker-free-online

National Center for Intensive Intervention—Student Progress Monitoring Tool for Data Collection and Graphing
www.intensiveintervention.org/resource/student-progress-monitoring-tool-data-collection-and-graphing

Observechange.org—Formative Grapher
http://observechange.org/graph

wikiHow—Create a Graph in Excel
www.wikihow.com/Create-a-Graph-in-Excel

PRINT RESOURCES

Barton, E. E., & Reichow, B. (2012). Guidelines for graphing data with Microsoft® Office 2007™, Office 2010™, and Office for Mac™ 2008 and 2011. *Journal of Early Intervention, 34,* 129–150.

Dixon, M. R., Jackson, J. W., Small, S. L., Horner-King, M. J., Lik, N. M. K., Garcia, Y., & Rosales, R. (2009). Creating single-subject design graphs in Microsoft Excel™ 2007. *Journal of Applied Behavior Analysis, 42,* 277–293.

Lo, Y. Y., & Konrad, M. (2007). A field-tested task analysis for creating single-subject graphs using Microsoft® Office Excel. *Journal of Behavioral Education, 16,* 155–189.

Riley-Tillman, T. C., & Burns, M. K. (2009). *Evaluating educational interventions: Single-case design for measuring response to intervention.* New York: Guilford Press.

Vanselow, N. R., & Bourret, J. C. (2012). Online interactive tutorials for creating graphs with Excel 2007 or 2010. *Behavior Analysis in Practice, 5,* 40–46. Retrieved from *www.abainternational.org/journals/behavior-analysis-in-practice/supplemental-materials.aspx.*

Zaslofsky, A. F., & Volpe, R. J. (2010). Graphing single-case data in Microsoft Excel™ 2007. *School Psychology Forum, 4,* 15–24. Retrieved from *www.nasponline.org/publications/spf/spfissues.aspx.*

in Figure 4.1). In these cases, time (i.e., dates, sessions) is plotted on the horizontal axis (i.e., the *X*-axis) and the extent of the variable of interest (e.g., adherence, quality, or exposure) is plotted on the vertical axis (i.e., the *Y*-axis). As needed, add phase-change lines—vertical lines added to a graph to indicate a change in phases (e.g., when changes were made to an intervention, when implementation support was provided, when relevant changes occurred in the implementation context; see example in Figure 4.1). Phase-change lines facilitate accurate interpretation of the data by indicating when data might not be directly comparable and when a change in data might be expected. A line graph is a useful and effective way to share data. Line graphs are easy to understand and, as such, can be valuable for communicating intervention fidelity to the implementer and for highlighting trends (i.e., patterns over time) that are useful for data interpretation and analysis.

Bar graphs are a helpful way to illustrate a comparison across different variables, such as the intervention fidelity of specific intervention steps (see example in Figure 4.2). When graphing intervention step fidelity, the horizontal axis represents intervention steps, and the vertical axis represents the percentage of intervention fidelity. Bar graphs can illustrate specific patterns of intervention steps that are implemented very consistently, less consistently, or not at all, which may not be clear when looking at a line graph that summarizes overall levels of intervention fidelity. Data displayed on a bar graph, such as intervention steps, are easily comparable because the relationships among the bars and the number value corresponding to each bar are clear.

Case Example

Ms. Rodriguez makes three graphs to summarize Mr. Suen's implementation. First, she makes a line graph that shows the intervention session fidelity adherence and quality of data across days. Second, she makes another line graph that shows the amount of time that the students are exposed to the Good Behavior Game. That is, she charts the number of minutes the game is played for each day it is implemented. Last, she makes a bar graph that depicts the percentage of game sessions each intervention step is implemented.

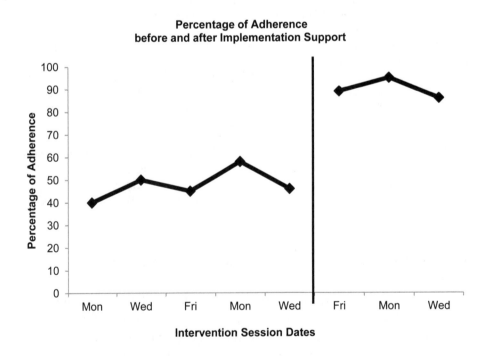

FIGURE 4.1. Sample line graph.

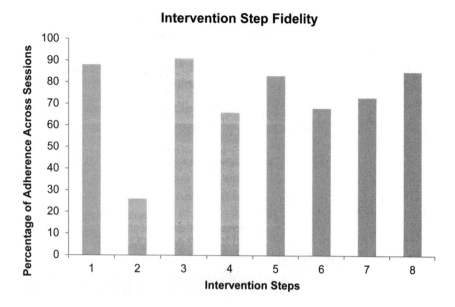

FIGURE 4.2. Sample bar graph.

Step 3: Interpret Graphs

After data have been graphed, it is time for interpretation. For intervention fidelity data, you want to know if intervention fidelity is sufficient to support learner outcomes. To interpret the graphed data, use visual analysis. Visual analysis is a systematic way of examining a graph to identify patterns and evaluate change (Horner et al., 2005; Riley-Tillman & Burns, 2009; Kratochwill et al., 2010). Although visual analysis can include many aspects of interpretation (see resources in Quick Tip 4.2 on p. 54 for more information), we suggest that your initial review of graphs include level, trend, and variability.

Level is the average value of the measured outcome (e.g., mean of intervention fidelity) within a phase (Kratochwill et al., 2010). As such, the level will provide an overall estimate of how well the intervention is being delivered (e.g., less than 30%, above 90%). You might expect a change in the level of intervention fidelity after providing an implementation support. Level can also be used to compare the extent of intervention fidelity across intervention steps in a bar graph. In Figure 4.3, a graph with a change in level is illustrated on the top, whereas a graph with no change in level is illustrated on the bottom. *Trend* is the pattern of change in the data over the course of time (Kratochwill et al., 2010). Trend will either be increasing, decreasing, or not present (i.e., flat). In Figure 4.4, the top graph illustrates an increasing trend, the middle graph illustrates a decreasing trend, and the bottom graph illustrates a data path without a trend. After initial intervention delivery, there is often a decreasing trend in intervention fidelity (e.g., Noell et al., 1997; Sanetti et al., 2015). That is, even when intervention fidelity data begin at a high level, a decreasing trend indicates it is lowering across time and can suggest that implementation support is needed. On the other hand, after providing implementation support, an increasing trend would be expected. *Variability* is the amount of "bounce" of data (i.e., the spread of data above and below the average; Kratochwill et al., 2010). When intervention fidelity data show

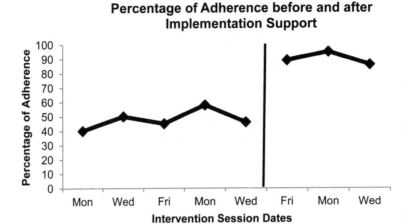

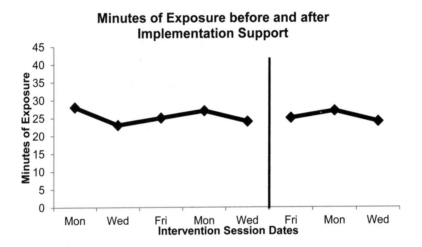

FIGURE 4.3. Graphs that illustrate a change in level and no change in level.

a relatively large amount of variability, it indicates that the intervention is being delivered inconsistently. When intervention fidelity data are variable, the learner is unlikely to benefit from the intervention, even if some of the individual data points are relatively high. In Figure 4.5, a graph illustrates data with substantial variability initially and, following a phase change, less variability.

Case Example

Ms. Rodriguez reviews the graphs to evaluate the level, trend, and variability of the data. She notes that Mr. Suen's adherence has been decreasing over time, and his quality has become more variable. That said, he consistently delivers the intervention for 30 minutes a day. Reviewing the intervention step bar graph, Ms. Rodriguez sees that Mr. Suen delivers some intervention steps consistently (e.g., announces the start of the game, tallies misbehaviors), but fails to deliver other steps (e.g., provide praise throughout the game, state winning team, provide reward).

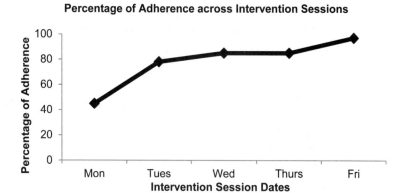

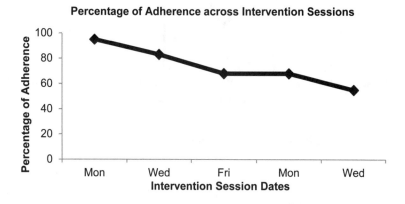

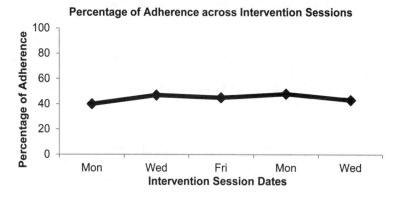

FIGURE 4.4. Graphs that illustrate increasing trend, decreasing trend, and no trend.

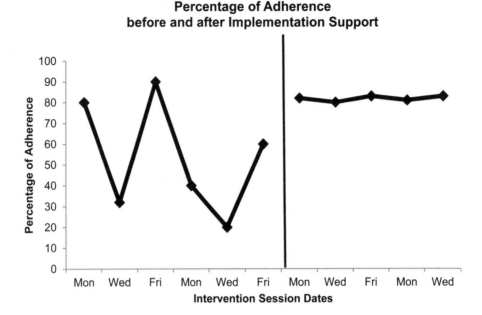

FIGURE 4.5. Graph illustrating variability.

Quick Tip 4.2. Visual Analysis Resources

Quick Tip Beyond trend, level, and variability, visual analysis can incorporate many more considerations to determine if the intervention has a functional relationship with the change, and it can summarize the effect of that intervention quantitatively. Although a thorough discussion is beyond the scope of this chapter, if interested, we encourage readers to refer to the following resources for further information.

INFORMATION ON VISUAL ANALYSIS

Cooper, J. O., Heron, T. E., & Heward, W. L. (2007). *Applied behavior analysis* (2nd ed.). Upper Saddle River, NJ: Pearson.

Kratochwill, T. R., Hitchcock, J., Horner, R. H., Levin, J. R., Odom, S. L., Rindskopf, D. M., & Shadish, W. R. (2010). Single-case designs technical documentation. In *What Works Clearinghouse: Procedures and standards handbook (version 2.0)*. Retrieved from *http://ies.ed.gov/ncee/wwc/pdf/wwc_procedures_v2_standards_handbook.pdf*.

Riley-Tillman, T. C., & Burns, M. (2009) *Evaluating educational interventions: Single-case designs for measuring response to intervention.* New York: Guilford Press.

Riley-Tillman, T. C., Burns, M. K., & Gibbons, K. (2013). *RTI applications: Vol. 2. Assessment analysis and decision making.* New York: Guilford Press.

Step 4: Develop a Summary Statement

To determine if intervention steps are being delivered sufficiently, develop a summary statement that (1) accounts for the trend, level, and variability of intervention fidelity across time; and (2) highlights specific intervention step fidelity. For example, a summary statement of session intervention fidelity data illustrated in Figure 4.6 might be described as the following: "Right after implementation began, the implementer demonstrated consistently high intervention fidelity, in the 90–95% adherence range [variability, level] with a flat trend [trend]. After 2 weeks, the implementer's intervention fidelity decreased over time [trend] to 40% adherence [level] and remained consistent [variability]." Although trend, level, and variability are most often associated with line graphs, these components can be applied to interpreting bar graphs, and a summary statement can be developed. For example, a summary statement of the bar graph of intervention steps fidelity illustrated in Figure 4.7 might be "The implementer consistently delivers consequence steps more often than antecedent steps [trend, variability], though the level of both types of steps is high (i.e., above 80%) [level]."

Based on your summary statement(s), decide whether intervention fidelity is sufficient to change learner outcomes. Research suggests that interventions need to be implemented at high levels (e.g., 80%, 90%, 100%) to result in changes for the learner (DiGennaro Reed et al., 2011; Noell et al., 1997; Sanetti et al., 2015; Wilder et al., 2006); however, there is no single criterion that divides sufficient from insufficient intervention fidelity (Gresham, 2014). **Intervention fidelity data need to be reviewed carefully to evaluate if (1) critical intervention steps are being implemented regularly, and (2) the extent of intervention fidelity is sufficient for the learner to make adequate progress.** If you are unsure whether intervention fidelity is sufficient, it is best to assume it is not, as, in most cases, implementa-

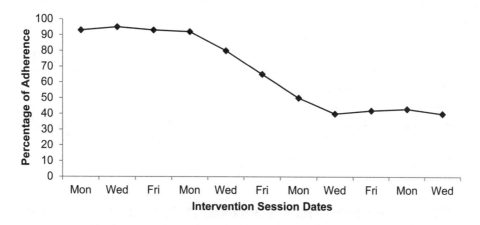

FIGURE 4.6. Summary statement graph. *Summary statement*: "Right after implementation began, the implementer demonstrated consistently high intervention fidelity, in the 90–95% adherence range [variability, level], with a flat trend [trend]. After 2 weeks, the implementer's intervention fidelity decreased over time [trend] to 40% adherence [level], and remained consistent [variability]."

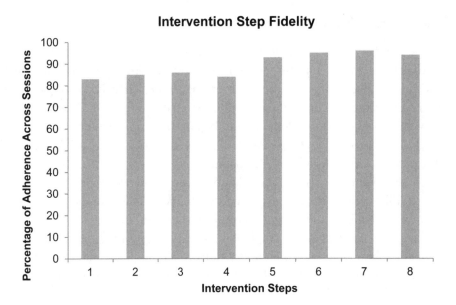

FIGURE 4.7. Summary statement graph. *Summary statement*: "The implementer consistently delivers consequence steps more often than antecedent steps [trend, variability], though the level of both types of steps is high (i.e., above 80%) [level]."

tion support should occur prior to changes in the learner intervention. Record the summary statements on the Data-Based Decision-Making Worksheet (in Appendix 4.1 at the end of the chapter).

Case Example

Ms. Rodriguez develops summary statements to describe the graphs and determine whether intervention fidelity seems sufficient. Since beginning the game, Mr. Suen's intervention integrity has been decreasing steadily from 90% adherence to 40% adherence. Although Mr. Suen's quality was initially moderate and stable (75–85%), it has become more variable over time (20–80%). Mr. Suen consistently plays the game for 30 minutes per day. His delivery of specific steps is variable, with some intervention steps delivered consistently (e.g., announces start of the game, tallies misbehaviors), but other steps variable or barely ever provided (e.g., provide praise throughout game, state winning team, provide reward). Based on the current patterns of implementation, Ms. Rodriguez thinks it is unlikely that student outcomes will improve, even though they are regularly exposed to the intervention.

DATA-BASED DECISION MAKING: INTEGRATE LEARNER OUTCOME AND INTERVENTION FIDELITY DATA

Now that you have graphed and interpreted the intervention fidelity data to identify whether intervention delivery is sufficient or insufficient, consider these findings along with learner

		Implementation Outcome	
		Sufficient Intervention Fidelity	**Insufficient Intervention Fidelity**
Intervention Outcome	**On Track to Meet Learner Goal**	*Data Profile A* The learner is making appropriate progress and the intervention is effective.	*Data Profile B* The learner is making appropriate progress, but it is unclear whether the intervention is effective.
	Not on Track to Meet Learner Goal	*Data Profile D* The learner is not making appropriate progress and the intervention may not be effective.	*Data Profile C* The learner is not making appropriate progress because the intervention has not been implemented as planned.

FIGURE 4.8. Using implementation and learner outcome data to identify a learner profile.

outcome data (Collier-Meek et al., 2013). Figure 4.8 illustrates how to link the intervention fidelity data with learner outcome data to identify the data profile that best describes the current status of learner progress and intervention delivery. Use the Data-Based Decision-Making Worksheet (Appendix 4.1) to walk through this process. Record the identified data profile on the Implementation Tracking Log (Appendix 2.1, pp. 30–31). Then refer to the specific data profile in the following material to learn about next steps.

Data Profile A: On Track to Meet Learner Goal and Sufficient Intervention Fidelity

Data Profile A suggests that the learner is making appropriate progress toward his or her intervention goal and that the intervention is being delivered as planned. Based on the learner's progress, the intervention can be considered effective. As such, it is not necessary to make any changes to the intervention or to the implementer's delivery at this time. The gist of the action steps that correspond to this scenario, described in the following mate-

---

Quick Tip 4.3. Using the Data-Based Decision-Making Worksheet and Data Profile Action Step Worksheets

We included several worksheets to guide you through data-based decision making and the next steps. These worksheets can be copied and used by you, the implementer, and other stakeholders. Keep the completed worksheets with the Implementation Tracking Log to note all of the activities completed to identify an intervention, implement and evaluate it, and provide support.

The Data-Based Decision-Making Worksheet in Appendix 4.1 includes space for recording the summary statements for intervention fidelity data and learner outcome data. Based on these summary statements, the worksheet prompts you to identify which data profile is indicated. If Data Profile A is indicated, note that the associated action steps are listed in this worksheet. If Data Profile B, C, or D is indicated, see the respective Data Profile Action Steps Worksheets in Appendices 4.2, 4.3, and 4.4. These worksheets include the action steps described within this chapter as well as space for recording the person responsible, due date, and any notes.

See Chapter 11 for case studies that illustrate the use of these worksheets in practice.

rial, is to continue the current plan to support the learner and implementer. Document your completion of these action steps using the Data-Based Decision-Making Worksheet (Appendix 4.1).

Data Profile A Action Steps

☐ Continue to deliver the intervention at its current level of intervention fidelity.

☐ Regularly evaluate learner outcome and intervention fidelity data to ensure that the current progress is maintained over time.

Data Profile B: On Track to Meet Learner Goal and Insufficient Intervention Fidelity

Data Profile B suggests that the learner is making appropriate progress toward his or her intervention goal, but the intervention is not being implemented as planned. In this case, it is unclear whether the intervention is effective. Although it is tempting to "leave well enough alone," it is worth doing some sleuthing to identify the cause of this surprising mismatch between the intervention and implementation outcomes.

There are at least three possible reasons for this pattern of intervention outcome and intervention fidelity data. **First, it may be necessary to update the intervention goal and the corresponding expected rate of learner progress.** The initial intervention goal may be an underestimate of what the learner could reasonably achieve. It is possible that if the intervention was delivered with even higher levels of intervention fidelity, the learner could reach even greater levels of improvement more quickly (e.g., Wilder et al., 2006). **Second, there may be issues with the intervention fidelity assessment method** (Perepletchikova & Kazdin, 2005). For example, the intervention fidelity tool may include several steps that are not functionally related to the improvements in learner outcomes, and if the implementer skipped these steps, it would result in a low intervention fidelity score. However, because the functionally related intervention steps are delivered consistently, there may be sufficient implementation to support learner outcomes. In another example, the intervention fidelity observations may not have accounted for implementation across the full session (e.g., day) and therefore may underestimate intervention fidelity. **Third, it is possible that something outside of the intervention is related to the improvement in learner outcomes.** For example, it is possible that a seemingly unrelated change in or outside of the implementation context (e.g., new teaching strategy, change in parent schedule, other outside support) may have led to improvements. If something outside the intervention is the cause of the improvement, it may be possible to fade or remove the intervention. This might be a welcome change, as it would reduce the amount of responsibilities for both the implementer and you, while still maintaining improvements for the learner. However, it is important to identify the supports that are responsible for the improvement in learner outcomes, and confirm that they are going to be maintained, prior to fading or removing the intervention.

The action steps that correspond to Data Profile B, described in the following material, involve identifying the reason for the pattern of intervention outcome and intervention fidelity data and then taking the corresponding next steps. Document your completion of these action steps using the Data Profile B Action Steps Worksheet (Appendix 4.2).

Data Profile B Action Steps

☐ Review research on the intervention to evaluate if the initial projection for the intervention goal was appropriate.

☐ Review the intervention step fidelity data, coverage of the intervention fidelity assessment method, and the representativeness of the observation sessions to identify if the intervention steps directly related to improvements in learner outcomes were appropriately captured. Note: It may be useful to review intervention research to identify what steps most impact learner outcomes.

☐ Talk with the implementer and other stakeholders (e.g., teacher, parent, paraprofessional, learner) to identify if any changes have been made outside of the intervention.

☐ Decide which of the three possible reasons for the data pattern most likely explains the current data profile. If the data profile is explained by reason 1, review the intervention goal and adjust the aim line for learner outcomes. Reevaluate the intervention outcome and intervention fidelity data to make an appropriate, data-driven decision about next steps. Continue to regularly evaluate learner outcome and intervention fidelity data.

☐ If the data profile is explained by reason 2, adjust the intervention fidelity assessment method and/or observation sessions to appropriately account for the intervention. Reevaluate the learner outcome and intervention fidelity data to make an appropriate, data-driven decision about next steps. Continue to regularly evaluate learner outcome and intervention fidelity data.

☐ If data profile is explained by reason 3, systematically discontinue implementation of the intervention, as intervention delivery may not be necessary for the learner to reach his or her goal. Continue to regularly evaluate learner outcome data to ensure that the improved outcomes are maintained.

Data Profile C: Not on Track to Meet Learner Goal and Insufficient Intervention Fidelity

Data Profile C suggests that the learner is not making enough progress to meet his or her intervention goal and the intervention is not being delivered sufficiently. In this case, intervention fidelity should be promoted through the delivery of an implementation support (Collier-Meek et al., 2013). **To identify the appropriate implementation support, (1) consider implementation history, (2) review intervention fidelity data to evaluate whether the issue is best characterized as a skill or performance deficit, and (3) consider relevant strategies and select one that is appropriate for the implementer and the context.**

Consider implementation history by reviewing the Implementation Tracking Log (Appendix 2.1, pp. 30–31) to review the implementation supports that have been provided previously to support the implementer and how long ago these supports were delivered.

Review the Fidelity Data Sheets for each implementation support that has been previously provided to make sure it was completed as designed (see Quick Tip 4.4 on p. 61 for more information). We recommend that prior to the delivery of an intervention, implementation planning (Chapter 5) and direct training (Chapter 6) be provided to adapt the intervention to the context in which it will be delivered and to give the implementer an opportunity to learn and practice the intervention. If these supports have not yet been provided, we suggest that you deliver both to facilitate higher levels of intervention fidelity (e.g., Collier-Meek et al., 2016). If these supports have been provided, but specific intervention steps are regularly missed, consider providing a targeted "booster" session of direct training, updating the implementation plan for those steps, or both. If implementation planning and direct training have been provided relatively recently or if intervention fidelity does not change after their delivery, consider another implementation support.

To identify an appropriate type of implementation support, review intervention fidelity data to identify whether the current implementation problem is more likely a skill or performance deficit. A skill deficit is present if the implementer is not able to deliver specific intervention steps or the entire intervention correctly or fluently (Duhon, Noell, Witt, & Freeland, 2004). An intervention fidelity issue is best characterized as a skill-based deficit if (1) intervention step fidelity data indicate that some steps are not implemented or (2) session intervention fidelity indicate low levels of quality, even if adherence is overall adequate. The implementation supports designed to address skill deficits include direct training, participant modeling, and role play. To decide among these implementation supports, see Table 4.2 for a description of these supports and some relevant considerations, review the brief summaries in Chapter 2, read the relevant implementation support strategy chapters, and

TABLE 4.2. Implementation Supports Designed to Address Skill Deficits

Implementation support	Description	Considerations
Direct training	Includes didactic training, consultant demonstration of the intervention, implementer practice, and feedback	• Most basic form of implementation support for a skill deficit • Recommended for all implementers prior to delivering the intervention, but may not be sufficient for some implementers
Participant modeling	Includes demonstration and practice of the intervention steps in the target environment	• Provides an opportunity to demonstrate implementation in the target environment • It may not always be possible (or acceptable to the implementer) to join the target environment
Role play	Includes review and practice of how to deliver an intervention through enacting several scenarios	• Provides an opportunity to practice challenging intervention scenarios • Practice may not sufficiently resemble real-time intervention delivery

Quick Tip 4.4. Completing Implementation Support Intervention Fidelity Forms

Just as monitoring the delivery of learner interventions is important, monitoring the delivery of implementation supports is necessary as well. During a conversation with an implementer, it is possible to miss one or a few steps (adherence) when discussing an intervention, to deliver a step in an awkward manner (quality), or to rush through the strategy (exposure). Evaluating intervention fidelity will ensure that you get a chance to review how well (or not) that you delivered the implementation support. That is why we included Fidelity Data Sheets for each implementation support, which you should complete after each session with the implementer. In most cases, you will self-report your own adherence, quality, and exposure, although sometimes you might have another person who is attending the meeting rate your intervention fidelity. The Fidelity Data Sheets are part of the implementation support guides, which you will use to guide your delivery of the strategies. When you complete these forms, you will rate and summarize adherence, quality, and exposure as follows:

ADHERENCE

To indicate if all of the key objectives of each step were delivered as designed, you will rate adherence on the following scale. Then you will sum the ratings across steps and calculate a total percentage of adherence. This percentage will indicate how many steps were completed as designed.

2 = All components of step delivered.
1 = Some components of step delivered.
0 = No components of step delivered.

QUALITY

To indicate how well each step was delivered, you will rate the quality on the following scale. Then you will sum the ratings across steps and calculate a total percentage of quality. This percentage will indicate how many steps were completed skillfully.

2 = Step delivered in a smooth, natural manner, responsive to the implementer, and with appropriate nonverbal interaction.
1 = Step delivered with some aspects of quality.
0 = Step delivered without any aspects of quality.

EXPOSURE

The top of each Implementation Support Guide includes space for the session start and end times. There is no required duration for any implementation support; however, it can be helpful to review how long the strategy lasted to ensure that it was completed in a reasonable time frame.

consider the implementer and the context. For example, some implementers may welcome you into their classroom or home during intervention implementation (necessary for participant modeling), whereas others would prefer to practice in a meeting format (i.e., role play).

A performance deficit is present if the implementer knows how to deliver the intervention, but is not doing so consistently (Duhon et al., 2004). An intervention fidelity issue is best characterized as a performance-based deficit if (1) intervention fidelity is inconsistent (e.g., fully implemented some days, low levels of intervention fidelity other days); (2) intervention fidelity has been high, but has decreased or become more variable over time; or (3) intervention fidelity data indicate low levels of exposure, even if adherence is overall adequate. The implementation supports designed to address performance deficits include implementation planning, self-monitoring, motivational interviewing, and performance feedback. To decide among these implementation supports, see Table 4.3 for a description of the supports and some relevant considerations, review the brief summaries in Chapter 2, read the relevant implementation support strategy chapters, and consider the implementer and his or her feedback about the intervention and its implementation. For example, if the implementer does not see the benefit of the intervention or of consistent intervention

TABLE 4.3. Implementation Supports Designed to Address Performance Deficits

Implementation support	Description	Considerations
Implementation planning	Detailed review of how to integrate delivering intervention steps into current routines and proactively address potential barriers	• Low-resource implementation support • Can be provided before or during intervention delivery
Self-monitoring	Have implementer monitor and evaluate his or her own intervention fidelity per jointly set goals	• Low-resource implementation support • Some implementers may not be amenable to self-monitoring
Motivational interviewing	Review the intervention and data in a supportive manner to highlight the relationship between changes in learner outcomes and consistent intervention fidelity	• Suited for an implementer who is not convinced that the intervention or sufficient intervention fidelity will make a difference • May be a challenging implementation support for some consultants
Performance feedback	Review intervention fidelity and learner outcome data with implementer, discuss any issues, and obtain commitment to higher levels of intervention fidelity	• Relatively brief strategy; however, it is recommended to be delivered regularly • Provides accountability for intervention fidelity

fidelity, motivational interviewing may be well suited, whereas if the implementer needs support in being held accountable for intervention delivery, self-monitoring or performance feedback may be best.

The action steps that correspond to Data Profile C, listed in the following material, involve reviewing implementation support history, determining whether the intervention fidelity data suggest a skill- or performance-based deficit, and then identifying and delivering an appropriate implementation support. Document your completion of these action steps using the Data Profile C Action Steps Worksheet (Appendix 4.3).

Data Profile C Action Steps

☐ Review implementation support history (Implementation Tracking Log in Appendix 2.1, pp. 30–31) to see if implementation planning and/or direct training have been provided recently. If these supports have not been delivered recently, consider providing one or both again.

☐ Evaluate intervention fidelity data to identify whether an implementer is struggling with a skill or a performance deficit.

☐ To identify a specific strategy, review relevant skill- or performance-deficit strategies and contextual and implementer factors.

☐ Prepare to deliver the implementation support by reading the appropriate chapter. Update the Implementation Tracking Log (Appendix 2.1, pp. 30–31).

☐ Continue to regularly evaluate implementation fidelity and learner outcome data.

Data Profile D: Not on Track to Meet Learner Goal and Sufficient Intervention Fidelity

Data Profile D suggests that the learner is not making sufficient progress to meet his or her intervention goal; however, intervention fidelity data show that the intervention is being implemented as planned. It appears that the intervention is not effective in helping the specific learner achieve his or her intervention goal.

Before changing the intervention, consider whether the intervention fidelity data accurately account for current implementation. The assessment method or sessions observed may have inadvertently suggested a higher level of implementation than actually occurred on a regular basis (Sanetti & Collier-Meek, 2014). For example, during the sessions observed, the implementer could have delivered the intervention with higher intervention fidelity than when not being observed, or the implementer could have overestimated his or her intervention fidelity on a self-report tool (e.g., Noell et al., 2005). Also, it will be important to consider varied dimensions of intervention fidelity. It is possible that all or most of the intervention steps are being delivered (i.e., adherence), but without enthusiasm (i.e., quality) and/or for an insufficient amount of time (i.e., exposure; Sanetti & Fallon, 2011). It may also be that particular intervention steps that are not consistently implemented are highly important to learner outcomes (Gresham, 2014). Thus, it is essential to carefully review intervention step fidelity. For example, if most of a token economy intervention is implemented (i.e., learner receives tokens throughout the day for appropriate behavior), but a step such as providing the reward is not delivered regularly, then the frequency of reinforcement may not be sufficient for the learner to change his or her behavior. A careful review of the intervention fidelity data may reveal that the intervention is not being consistently or comprehensively delivered, even despite initial impressions that intervention fidelity was sufficient (Pereplet-chikova & Kazdin, 2005).

If further review of intervention fidelity data indicates that an intervention is being sufficiently delivered, it may be appropriate to modify the learner's intervention (Codding & Lane, 2015). For instance, you could systematically increase the intensity of the intervention. That is, you could increase the frequency and/or duration of the intervention (e.g., delivering an academic intervention four times per week instead of two) or change the format of intervention delivery to decrease the ratio of learners to teachers (e.g., delivering an academic intervention to a learner one-to-one rather than in a small group; Codding & Lane, 2015). Make modifications to the intervention that are research supported and theoretically sound.

If modifications to the intensity of the intervention are not appropriate or do not result in improvements for the learner, it may be necessary to change the identified intervention (Collier-Meek et al., 2013). In this case, go back to the beginning of the problem-solving process to review the baseline data, reconsider the hypotheses developed, and identify an alternative evidence-based intervention (Kratochwill et al., 2014).

The action steps that correspond to Data Profile D, listed in the following material, involve identifying the reason for the pattern of learner outcome and intervention fidelity data and then taking corresponding next steps. Document your completion of these action steps using the Data Profile D Action Steps Worksheet (Appendix 4.4).

Data Profile D Action Steps

☐ Make sure the intervention fidelity data accurately capture the intervention. To do so, review the intervention step fidelity data, intervention fidelity assessment method, and the representativeness of the observations session. Note: It may be useful to review intervention research to identify which steps most impact learner outcomes. If appropriate, revise the intervention fidelity assessment method. Reevaluate the learner outcome and intervention fidelity data to make an appropriate, data-driven decision about next steps.

☐ Consider increasing the intensity of the intervention. If such modifications are made, consider returning to implementation planning (Chapter 5) and/or direct training (Chapter 6) to ensure that the modifications are appropriate for the context and that the implementer is prepared to deliver the modified intervention. After subsequent implementation, evaluate the learner outcome and intervention fidelity data to make an appropriate, data-driven decision about next steps.

☐ Decide to change interventions. To do so, begin the problem-solving process again by reviewing learner outcome data to identify another evidence-based intervention.

Case Example

Ms. Rodriguez's review of the data indicated that intervention fidelity data were insufficient and student outcomes were poor; Data Profile C best described the status of this case. Ms. Rodriguez provided direct training before Mr. Suen began the next Good Behavior Game. She needed to determine whether Mr. Suen's challenges with implementation were more attributed to a skill or performance deficit. Ms. Rodriguez reviewed Mr. Suen's data carefully and saw that he provided all intervention steps at least a few times, indicating that he did know how to deliver them. As such, she thought the situation was best characterized as a performance deficit and determined that she would provide self-monitoring instruction to help Mr. Suen keep track of his intervention fidelity and increase the likelihood that he consistently delivered the Good Behavior Game.

SUMMARY

This chapter addressed how to evaluate intervention fidelity and integrate it with learner outcome data to make data-based decisions about the need for implementation support. The process of evaluating intervention fidelity data involves summarizing, graphing, interpreting, and developing a summary statement to determine whether there is sufficient or insufficient implementation. Then, one of four data profiles can be identified when intervention and implementation data are reviewed together (Collier-Meek et al., 2013). Depending on whether the learner is on track to meet his or her goal and intervention fidelity is deemed sufficient or insufficient, the appropriate next step will involve continuing current practice, conducting further evaluation, providing implementation support, or changing the intervention. The case of Mr. Suen's implementation of the Good Behavior Game and Ms. Rodriguez's review of the intervention fidelity data illustrated the process here. For more examples, see Chapter 11.

Data-Based Decision-Making Worksheet

Learner: _____ Implementer: _____

Consultant: _____ Date: _____

First, write the intervention fidelity summary statement: _____

_____

_____

_____

Check below to indicate whether intervention fidelity is sufficient or insufficient.

Next, write the learner outcome summary statement: _____

_____

_____

_____

Check below to indicate whether the learner is or is not on track to meet his or her goal.

Last, identify and circle the appropriate Data Profile. Record it on the Implementation Tracking Log (Appendix 2.1). Complete appropriate action steps (see Data Profile Action Steps Worksheets for Data Profiles B–D in the following appendices).

	☐ **Sufficient** Intervention Fidelity	☐ **Insufficient** Intervention Fidelity
☐ Learner **is** on track to meet his or her goal	*Data Profile A* The learner is making appropriate progress and the intervention is effective. ☐ Continue to deliver intervention at current level ☐ Regularly evaluate learner outcome and intervention fidelity data Date of next meeting: _____	*Data Profile B* The learner is making appropriate progress, but it is unclear whether the intervention is effective. ☐ See Data Profile B Action Steps Worksheet (Appendix 4.2)
☐ Learner **is not** on track to meet his or her goal	*Data Profile D* The learner is not making appropriate progress and the intervention may not be effective. ☐ See Data Profile C Action Steps Worksheet (Appendix 4.3)	*Data Profile C* The learner is not making appropriate progress because the intervention has not been implemented as planned. ☐ See Data Profile D Action Steps Worksheet (Appendix 4.4)

Data Profile B [+LO –IF] Action Steps Worksheet

Learner: _____   Implementer: _____   Consultant: _____   Intervention: _____

Action Steps	Person Responsible	Date Due	Notes
Review research on the intervention to evaluate if the initial projection for the intervention goal was appropriate.			
To identify if the intervention steps directly related to improvements in learner outcomes were appropriately captured, review . . . • the *intervention step fidelity data*, • coverage of the intervention fidelity assessment method, and • the representativeness of the *observation sessions*. • *Note:* It may be useful to review intervention research to identify which steps most impact learner outcomes.			
Talk with the implementer and other stakeholders (e.g., teacher, parent, paraprofessional, learner) to learn if any changes have been made outside of the intervention.			
Decide which of the three possible reasons for the data pattern most likely explains the current scenario. (see p. 58)			

(continued)

Data Profile B [+LO −IF] Action Steps Worksheet *(page 2 of 2)*

Action Steps	Person Responsible	Date Due	Notes
If the data profile is explained by reason 1: • *Review the intervention goal* and adjust the aim line for learner outcomes. • *Reevaluate the intervention outcome and intervention fidelity data* to make an appropriate, data-driven decision about next steps. • Continue to *regularly evaluate learner outcome and intervention fidelity data.*			
If the data profile is explained by reason 2: • *Adjust the intervention fidelity assessment method and/or observation sessions* to appropriately account for the intervention. • *Reevaluate the learner outcome and intervention fidelity data* to make an appropriate, data-driven decision about next steps. • Continue to *regularly evaluate learner outcome and intervention fidelity data.*			
If the data profile is explained by reason 3: • *Systematically discontinue implementation* of the intervention, as it may not be necessary for the learner to reach his or her goal. • Continue to *regularly evaluate learner outcome data* to ensure that the improved outcomes are maintained.			

Data Profile C [–LO –IF] Action Steps Worksheet

Learner: _____   Implementer: _____   Consultant: _____   Intervention: _____

Action Steps	Person Responsible	Date Due	Notes
Review *implementation support history* (Implementation Tracking Log in Appendix 2.1). • See if *implementation planning and/or direct training* has been provided recently. • If these supports have not been delivered recently, *consider providing one or both again.*			
Evaluate *intervention fidelity data* to identify whether an implementer is struggling with a skill or performance deficit. • *Skill deficit*—implementer is not able to deliver intervention steps skillfully or fluently. • *Performance deficit*—implementer knows how to deliver the intervention, but struggles to do so consistently.			
To *identify a specific strategy*, review relevant skill- or performance-deficit strategies and contextual and implementer factors.			
Prepare *to deliver the implementation support.* • Read the appropriate chapter. • Complete the *preparation activities* outlined in the chapter.			
Deliver *the implementation support.* • Complete the *follow-up* activities outlined in the chapter. • Update the *Implementation Tracking Log* (Appendix 2.1).			
Continue to *regularly evaluate implementation fidelity and learner outcome data.*			

Data Profile D [–LO +IF] Action Steps Worksheet

Learner: _____   Implementer: _____   Consultant: _____   Intervention: _____

Action Steps	Person Responsible	Date Due	Notes

Make sure that the intervention fidelity data accurately captures the intervention.
• To identify if the intervention steps directly related to improvements in learner outcomes were appropriately captured, review . . .
  ○ the *intervention step fidelity data,*
  ○ coverage of the intervention fidelity *assessment method,* and
  ○ the representativeness of the *observation sessions.*
• Note: It may be useful to review intervention research to identify which steps most impact learner outcomes.
• If appropriate, *revise the intervention fidelity assessment method.*
• *Reevaluate the learner outcome and intervention fidelity data to make an appropriate, data-driven decision about next steps.*			

Consider increasing the intensity of the intervention. • If such modifications are made, consider *returning to implementation planning* (Chapter 5) *and/or direct training* (Chapter 6) to ensure that the modifications are appropriate for the context and that the implementer is prepared to deliver the intervention. • After subsequent implementation, *evaluate the learner outcome and intervention fidelity data* to make an appropriate, data-driven decision about next steps.			
Decide to change interventions. • To do so, *begin the problem-solving process again* by reviewing learner outcome data to identify another evidence-based intervention.			

PART III

IMPLEMENTATION SUPPORT STRATEGIES

CHAPTER 5

Implementation Planning

WHAT IS IMPLEMENTATION PLANNING?

Implementation planning is a form of implementation support that involves meeting with an implementer to increase his or her knowledge of how to deliver each step of an intervention and identify potential barriers to ongoing implementation (Box 5.1). Implementation planning includes two phases: (1) action planning, which involves planning the logistics of implementation; and (2) coping planning, which involves identifying barriers to implemen-

---

BOX 5.1. Implementation Planning Snapshot

SNAP SHOT

Who? All implementers.

What? A brief meeting to review intervention steps, offer an opportunity for planned adaptation of the intervention, explicitly define the logistics of intervention implementation, as well as identify and problem-solve possible barriers to implementation.

Where? When? Complete implementation planning in a private space immediately after initially introducing a new intervention to an implementer, and before training.

Why? Implementation planning increases implementer clarity about intervention steps, allows for adaptations to be made systematically to increase contextual fit, and proactively acknowledges and addresses the implementer's perceived barriers to implementation.

---

tation and developing strategies to overcome those barriers (see Figure 5.1). For the first step in action planning, you and the implementer review each intervention step and discuss if any adaptations are needed to increase the likelihood that it will be implemented with fidelity. Across human service fields, a majority of interventions are adapted when used in practice (Durlak & DuPre, 2008; Ringwalt et al., 2003). Implementation planning provides a process for systematically considering adaptations, accepting those that are not likely to decrease the effectiveness of the intervention, and documenting the adaptations so that the implementation of the adapted intervention can be evaluated.

Once any needed adaptations have been made, implementation planning involves discussing each intervention step and specifying *when, how often, for how long,* and *where* it will be implemented. The last step in planning implementation logistics involves identifying any resources that will be needed to implement each intervention step, who is responsible for obtaining each resource, and by when he or she will obtain it.

With action planning completed, coping planning begins. During coping planning, the implementer identifies the barriers he or she believes are most likely to arise and impede his or her implementation of the intervention. Once the implementer has identified up to four possible barriers, you and the implementer brainstorm ways to maintain intervention implementation in the presence of each of these barriers.

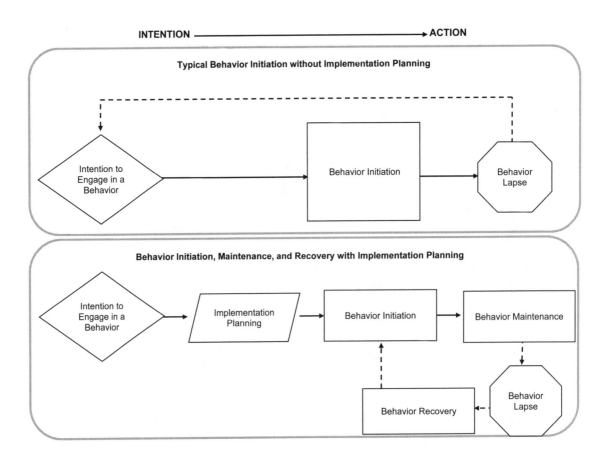

FIGURE 5.1. Behavior initiation with and without implementation planning.

RESEARCH ON IMPLEMENTATION PLANNING

Implementation planning has been found to be effective in both school and home settings to address a range of behavioral and academic concerns (Collier-Meek, Sanetti, et al., 2018; Fallon et al., 2016; Sanetti & Collier-Meek, 2015; Sanetti et al., 2015; Sanetti, Collier-Meek, Long, Kim, & Kratochwill, 2014; Sanetti, Williamson, Long, & Kratochwill, 2018). More specifically, several studies have demonstrated that implementation planning can effectively increase general education teachers' adherence and quality when implementing behavior support plans (Sanetti et al., 2014, 2015) and classroom management plans (Collier-Meek, Sanetti, et al., 2018; Sanetti & Collier-Meek, 2015; Sanetti et al., 2018). It also effectively increased special education teachers' implementation of a schoolwide behavior plan in an alternative school setting (Long, Sanetti, Lark, & Connolly, 2018) and parents' implementation of a home-based behavioral intervention (Fallon et al., 2016). In terms of academics, implementation planning effectively increased implementation of a math fluency intervention (Byron & Sanetti, 2018; Altschaefl & Kratochwill, 2016). These studies echo the results of decades of research in health psychology and suggest that logistical planning and barrier identification facilitate implementers' movement from having an intention to implement to maintaining implementation (e.g., Schwartzer, 2008; Scholz, Schüz, Ziegelmann, Lippke, & Schwarzer, 2008; Sniehotta, Scholz, & Schwarzer, 2005).

HOW DOES IMPLEMENTATION PLANNING WORK?

Implementation planning is based on the health action process approach (HAPA; Schwarzer, 1992, 2008), an empirically supported theory of adult behavior change that suggests that there are two stages to engaging in a new behavior. First, the individual has to develop an intention to change his or her behavior. In terms of implementing interventions, this typically requires the implementer to believe that (1) there is an issue that requires intervention, (2) he or she is capable of intervening, and (3) intervention implementation is likely to help. Second, the individual has to actually act on his or her intention and engage in the new behavior, and then maintain that behavior across time. Left to our own devices, the shift from the first stage to the second stage is where most of us get tripped up. The detailed logistical planning and barrier identification involved in implementation planning have been found to help people successfully move from having an intention to change their behavior to actually engaging in the new behavior (Schwarzer, 1992, 2008).

WHAT IMPLEMENTERS WILL BENEFIT FROM IMPLEMENTATION PLANNING?

Implementation planning can benefit any implementer. Given its focus, we recommend that you use implementation planning with all implementers when you introduce a new intervention. Because you and the implementer may adapt the intervention during this process, it is most efficient to complete implementation planning before embarking on direct training or other implementation support strategies. For interventions that are to be implemented across contexts or implementers (e.g., homeroom teachers, specialist teachers), it is most time efficient to complete implementation planning with all implementers present. This format will better equip you to adapt the intervention to fit in each of the contexts, and decrease barriers that may be unique to specific implementers or contexts. The combination of implementation planning and direct training will set up the implementers for successful implementation, which will save you time and energy in supporting them across time.

Implementation planning can also be used to increase implementation. If you have provided training to an implementer, but intervention fidelity data suggest that he or she is struggling to implement the intervention consistently across time, implementation planning can be an effective way to review the intervention plan, make adaptations to the plan that may increase feasibility, and problem-solve barriers to implementation.

GETTING READY FOR IMPLEMENTATION PLANNING

Implementation planning is a conversation-based implementation support strategy that requires some preparation ahead of time to allow for a smooth and productive session with the implementer. Getting ready to deliver implementation planning involves three steps, outlined in Box 5.2 and described below.

Step 1: Review the Intervention and Current Data

To prepare for implementation planning, review the intervention and current data, if available. Specifically, review the intervention plan. Once familiar, *break down the intervention plan so that you are able to clearly discuss the discrete steps of the intervention* (sometimes referred to as "components"). We are often asked if there is a "right way" to divide

---

BOX 5.2. Getting Ready to Deliver Implementation Planning

1. Review the intervention and current data.
   - Familiarize yourself with and break down the intervention plan.
   - If using implementation planning after implementation has already begun:
     ○ Review intervention goal and, using data, the learner's current progress.
     ○ Evaluate intervention fidelity data.
2. Prepare for implementation planning.
   - Read about implementation planning.
     ○ Prepare the Action and Coping Planning Worksheets.
     ○ Practice dialogue, as needed, to be comfortable in the meeting.
3. Identify session logistics.
   - Schedule implementation planning session.
   - Reach out to the implementer.
   - Bring implementation planning materials to the session.

an intervention into steps. For some interventions it is pretty clear, but for others, less so. The primary question you want to ask yourself is, "Are there steps that fit together or can be grouped in a logical way?" If so, plan to address those steps together, as a group, rather than in individual pieces.

Your goal is to divide the intervention plan into grouped steps that will help the implementer understand (1) how intervention steps are related to others in the group, (2) how groups of interventions steps are related to one another, and (3) the overall intervention plan. For a behavior support plan, it may be helpful to group intervention steps into antecedent (e.g., establishing and defining a classroom schedule, active supervision), teaching (e.g., teach behavioral expectations, teach problem solving), and consequence (e.g., classwide group contingencies, positive reinforcement) strategies. For other types of interventions, organize the steps into logical groups to discuss with the implementer. For example, you may divide the intervention steps according to when the steps must be implemented (e.g., all steps delivered at once, different steps provided at separate times) or in relation to the theoretical links between the steps (e.g., if several steps are based on one principle, if intervention steps build on one another).

If implementation planning is being used to proactively adapt an intervention prior to implementation, move on to Step 2 in the next section. If, however, you are using implementation planning to increase an implementer's intervention fidelity, *review the intervention goal and the learner's progress* and *review intervention fidelity data* so that you are comfortable describing current patterns in these data sources (e.g., level, trend, variability, relationship between data sources). If possible, make graphs to illustrate this information and thereby provide a rationale for why there is a need for the implementation planning session (see Chapter 4).

Step 2: Prepare for Implementation Planning

To be comfortable delivering this strategy, carefully *read about implementation planning* and familiarize yourself with the strategy steps and talking points (see Appendix 5.1). Confirm your understanding of the purpose of the strategy and each of the steps. To make the session with the implementer as efficient as possible, we recommend that you *prepare the Action and Coping Planning Worksheets* (Appendices 5.2A–52.D). Make copies of all the worksheets, and then complete the first and second columns of the Action Plan Worksheet, Part A (Appendix 5.2A), by writing the intervention components identified in Step 1. Having this portion filled in already will allow you to focus more of your attention on the implementer's concerns and needs as opposed to the completion of the worksheet. In addition to these worksheets, prepare any other necessary information or materials (e.g., graphs, reports, written intervention plan). To *practice your dialogue*, review the Implementation Planning Guide (Appendix 5.1), and if applicable, review intervention fidelity and outcome data. This preparation will help you to maximize the strategy session.

Step 3: Identify Session Logistics

Once ready, it is necessary to plan the session logistics. To *schedule implementation planning*, determine how long the meeting will last, when to hold the meeting, and how many

---

Quick Tip 5.1. Bring Extra Action and Coping Planning Worksheets

 To facilitate the meeting process, we highly recommend that you bring a second copy of the intervention plan and the Action and Coping Planning Worksheets so that the implementer can follow along. We have found that doing so helps implementers understand the questions and keeps the meeting moving at a relatively quick pace.

---

sessions are needed to complete the strategy. Plan to meet for approximately 30 minutes, although some implementation planning sessions may be shorter or longer. Decide who will be involved (e.g., primary implementer, potential collaborators). In some cases, there is more than one person implementing the intervention (e.g., paraprofessionals, school support professionals) or other stakeholders (e.g., case worker, parent) who may be interested in attending. Arrange where you will meet. You will need a quiet space that offers privacy for discussion. Make sure that the time and location are feasible for implementer. *Reach out to the implementer* ahead of the implementation planning session. If you think it would be helpful for the implementer to review any materials prior to the strategy meeting, provide those in advance (e.g., written list of intervention steps, sample intervention materials, research, data). *Bring implementation planning materials* to the session: the Implementation Planning Guide (Appendix 5.1), the written intervention plan, the Action Planning and Coping Planning Worksheets (Appendix 5.2), and, if applicable, graphs of intervention fidelity and learner outcome data.

IMPLEMENTATION PLANNING STEP-BY-STEP

Implementation planning involves reviewing the intervention, adapting intervention steps to the implementation context, and collaboratively developing an implementation plan during a meeting with the implementer. The 11 steps of a typical implementation planning session are listed in Box 5.3. The Implementation Planning Guide (Appendix 5.1) at the end of this chapter includes the key objectives and sample language for each step, as well as space for recording the implementer's responses. This guide can be copied and used for delivering this implementation support in your practice. A description of the steps involved in implementation planning, including key objectives and quick tips for delivery, are provided below.

Step 1: Explain the Purpose of the Session

- Provide an overview of implementation planning.
- Begin implementation planning in an open, supportive manner.

The purpose of this step is to open the implementation planning session in a collaborative manner by previewing the plan for the session, explaining implementation planning, and developing goals for the session. Start by providing a general description of why you are

> ## BOX 5.3. Implementation Planning Steps
>
> 1. Explain the purpose of the session.
> 2. Review the target concern and goal.
> 3. Review the intervention steps.
> 4. Modify the intervention steps, if needed.
> 5. Identify the logistics of each intervention step.
> 6. Discuss how needed resources may be obtained, if applicable.
> 7. Summarize the action plan.
> 8. Identify potential barriers to implementation.
> 9. Identify potential strategies to address barriers.
> 10. Summarize coping planning.
> 11. Review the meeting and thank the implementer.

meeting with the implementer, explaining that you are going to consider the intervention logistics and plan for implementation.

Explain to the implementer that implementation planning consists of two stages. The goal of the first stage is for the consultant and the implementer to look at the intervention steps and plan the details of the intervention. The goal of the second stage is to identify and problem-solve any barriers to implementation. Thus, the overall purpose of implementation planning is to facilitate the definition and adaptation of the intervention so that it fits the implementer's specific context.

Work with the implementer to collaboratively develop goals for the session, as doing so will allow you to target the discussion and ensure that there is a shared vision for the meeting. Goals for implementation planning might include helping the implementer prepare for the implementation or making adaptations to the intervention to ensure that it is contextually appropriate. Use your understanding of the implementation planning strategy to help target the implementer's suggestions for the session goals. Once you've decided on shared goals, briefly explain how implementation planning will help meet these session goals.

Step 2: Review the Target Concern and Goal

- Review the target concern, current data, and intervention goal.
- Describe generally how the intervention can address the learner's issue and support the learner to meet his or her goal.

To set up the discussion of the intervention, briefly review the target concern for the learner, current learner outcome data (if available), and the intervention goal. That is, you may highlight the major concerns and address the current level of progress compared to the intervention goal. This review of the target concern will ensure that the discussion of the intervention through the rest of the implementation planning steps is appropriately contextualized.

Step 3: Review the Intervention Steps

- Show the implementer the list of intervention steps (on Action Plan Worksheet, Part A).
- Discuss if the organization of intervention steps makes sense to the implementer; if not, revise.

This is the first step of action planning, and it consists of reviewing the list of intervention steps with the implementer (see Action Plan Worksheet, Part A, Appendix 5.2A). If the intervention steps have been grouped together, as recommended above, it is important for you to go over how the steps were grouped and the logic behind the grouping, to make sure that the steps are divided in a way that makes sense to the implementer. If the implementer has any questions or suggestions about how the steps have been organized, make revisions to the list of intervention steps at this time. When reviewing the intervention, make sure that what each step requires is clear and, if helpful, briefly describe why each step is important to the outcomes.

Step 4: Modify the Intervention Steps, If Needed

- Ask the implementer if modifications to intervention steps could increase feasibility or contextual fit.
- Keep in mind the empirical and theoretical support for any modifications to intervention steps.

It is important to ensure that the intervention is feasible and contextually appropriate. At this point, ask if the implementer has identified any intervention steps that may need modifications to be appropriate for his or her context or the learner. If modifications are requested, it is important to keep in mind the empirical and theoretical support for each intervention step and to ensure that any revisions follow the same theoretical logic. Have an active discussion that results in an evidence-based intervention that is well suited to the implementer's context. Any modifications that are made should be agreed upon by the consultant and the implementer, and recorded on the Action Plan Worksheet, Part A (Appendix 5.2A).

Step 5: Identify the Logistics of Each Intervention Step

- Discuss how proactively planning logistics of an intervention can help implementation.
- Ask the implementer to identify logistics of implementation and needed resources.
- Record implementer responses regarding intervention logistics on Action Plan Worksheet, Part B (Appendix 5.2B).

The purpose of this step is to plan out the logistical aspects of the intervention. Planning exactly what is needed to accomplish each step of the intervention plan facilitates sustained implementation of the plan. For each intervention step, the consultant and implementer should work together to answer the following questions:

- **When?** When will this step of the intervention plan be completed? For steps occurring daily, this may mean a particular time of day (e.g., 9:00 A.M.) or a particular time period (e.g., during the morning meeting, during the fifth class period). For steps that occur only as needed, the type of behavior occurring prior to the step (i.e., the antecedent) can be described. Examples of this option may include "when students are off task" or "when students are showing appropriate behavior." Some steps may include permanent products (e.g., posting a schedule, arranging the classroom in a way that minimizes crowding and distraction) and may only need to be completed once. For steps such as these, examples may include "At the beginning of the year" or "By next Tuesday."

- **How often?** How often will this step of the intervention be completed? Examples may include "daily" or "as needed." You may want to use this step to specify a goal for how often this step should be delivered. For example, behavior-specific praise could be described as being provided "at least 10 times per period." For steps involving simple permanent products, such as posting behavioral expectations, "Once at the beginning of the year" may be appropriate.

- **For how long?** For how long will this intervention step last? Examples may include a specific length of time for more discrete steps (e.g., 5 minutes, 20 minutes). Some steps may not have a proscribed length of time to complete, and "as needed" may be appropriate. Steps involving one act that results in implementation across time (e.g., posting behavioral expectations in the classroom) may last all year.

- **Where?** Where will this intervention step occur? For school-based interventions, many (if not most) intervention steps may occur within the classroom. However, it may be appropriate to describe a specific place in the classroom (e.g., on the rug, on the calendar board, at the teacher's desk) where each intervention step will occur. Likewise, consider if the intervention will be implemented across multiple school settings (e.g., hallway, bus, physical education, library). For home- or community-based interventions, specifying all possible locations where an intervention will take place is essential to considering feasibility, possible adaptations across settings, and needed resources, which could be different across all settings.

- **Resources needed?** What resources or materials (if any) are needed to complete this step? Examples of resources may include paper and pencil, materials for a specific lesson, or supplies for a reinforcement system (see Appendix 5.2C).

All of these responses can be listed on the Action Plan Worksheet, Part B (Appendix 5.2B). If the implementer struggles to identify the logistics of implementation, the Action Plan Sample Responses form (Appendix 5.2D) can be used to provide examples. It can also be helpful to ask questions such as "What would that step look like?" or "Talk me through the completion of that step." These types of questions may help elicit responses from the implementer about how each step of the intervention will be completed. It is important to ensure that the implementer's responses reflect his or her impressions of how the intervention will work in his or her context.

Step 6: Discuss How Needed Resources May Be Obtained, If Applicable

- Identify how, when, and by whom needed resources can be obtained.
- Record plan for obtaining resources on Action Plan Worksheet, Part C.

If additional materials are needed for the intervention steps, identify how those materials can be accessed. Is the implementer able to obtain them? Can you provide them or develop them, if necessary? Do others (e.g., an administrator or other professional) need to be approached to obtain the materials? In thinking about how to access materials, keep in mind that the quicker these resources are obtained, the faster the intervention can be implemented. If necessary resources cannot be obtained quickly, the implementation of the intervention may be delayed. Make sure to delineate what resources are needed, who is responsible for obtaining them, and by when the resources will be obtained on Action Plan Worksheet, Part C (Appendix 5.2C).

Step 7: Summarize the Action Plan

- Summarize revisions made (if applicable) and the logistical details of implementation.
- Praise the implementer for his or her participation in the process.

Review and summarize any revisions that have been made to the intervention plan and the logistical details that were determined for each intervention step. Summarizing the plan ensures that you and the implementer are on the same page about the action plan. Once the action plan has been reviewed, you should praise the implementer for participating in the process. This step completes the action planning process.

Step 8: Identify Potential Barriers to Implementation

- Ask the implementer to identify major anticipated or current barriers to intervention implementation.
- Ask the implementer to prioritize his or her top four barriers.
- Record barriers on Coping Plan Worksheet.

This is the first step in the Coping Planning process. First, you should show the implementer the Coping Plan Worksheet (Appendix 5.2E) and ask for any major anticipated or current barriers to implementing the intervention as outlined in the action plan. Make sure the barriers are identified by the implementer and thus reflect his or her issues with consistently delivering the intervention with high levels of intervention fidelity. Barriers may be related to intervention (e.g., remembering many new steps, implementing particularly challenging steps), the learner (e.g., strained relationship with the learner, being unsure if the learner will like the intervention), implementation (e.g., having sufficient time for preparation, managing the new responsibility), or context (e.g., how to support other individuals while engaging in implementation, having a supervisor who doesn't understand the

---

Quick Tip 5.2. Identifying Implementation Barriers

 Some implementers may have difficulty coming up with barriers on their own. In this case, it can be helpful to provide the implementer with an example of a barrier related to a different intervention. For example, if the implementer is implementing an academic intervention, it would be appropriate to provide an example from a behavioral intervention. If the intervention targets one student, it may be appropriate to provide an example from an intervention that targets multiple students or an entire classroom.

---

importance of the intervention). Have the implementer rank up to four barriers in order of importance (1 = highest priority, 2 = second highest, etc.).

Step 9: *Identify Potential Strategies to Address Barriers*

- Brainstorm ways to maintain implementation in the presence of each barrier.
- Write identified strategies on the Coping Plan Worksheet.

Once barriers have been identified, problem-solve how to overcome them. Ask the implementer to brainstorm ways that the intervention can be maintained in the presence of each of the top four barriers. If the implementer struggles to identify strategies, provide suggestions or ideas in a collaborative manner. When identifying strategies, consider potential modifications to the intervention or implementation context (e.g., modifying implementer's other responsibilities, eliciting available support) as well as suggestions related to prompting and reinforcing implementation. For example, if the implementer has identified lack of time as an implementation barrier, work with him or her to identify possible ways to make the intervention or specific intervention steps more efficient or to reduce other responsibilities. Or, as is the case with the implementation of many behavioral interventions, you can describe how the intervention may save the implementer time if implemented effectively. For example, a behavior intervention designed to reduce or prevent challenging behaviors will, if effective, reduce the amount of time the implementer spends managing those behaviors. Once an appropriate strategy has been identified to address a barrier, it should be written on the Coping Plan Worksheet (Appendix 5.2E).

Step 10: *Summarize Coping Planning*

- Summarize the strategies identified to address barriers.
- Praise the implementer for his or her participation in the process.

This is the last step in the coping planning process. Summarize the strategies that have been developed to overcome the identified barriers to implementation. Confirm that the implementer believes that these strategies will help address the barriers. Next, praise the implementer for his or her participation in the coping planning process.

Step 11: Review the Meeting and Thank the Implementer

- Review the meeting discussion and decisions.
- Thank the implementer and close the meeting.

To complete this last step, review the process of implementation planning and ask the implementer if he or she has any questions related to (1) the revisions made to the intervention plan (if applicable), (2) the logistics of implementation, (3) who is responsible for obtaining any needed resources and by when this will be accomplished, and/or (4) the identified barriers and related strategies to maintain implementation. Once all questions have been answered, inform the implementer that you will provide a clean, typed copy of the implementation plan and obtain any resources for which you are responsible. Finally, thank the implementer for his or her time and work during the implementation planning process.

FOLLOW-UP AFTER IMPLEMENTATION PLANNING

To cement the discussion and the progress made during implementation planning, we suggest that you engage in some activities after the session. Follow-up after implementation planning involves five steps, outlined in Box 5.4 and described below.

Review session notes to ensure that the strategy was delivered as planned. To do so, check the Implementation Planning Guide (Appendix 5.1) and complete a self-assessment using the Fidelity Data Sheet for Implementation Planning (Appendix 5.3) to see if you addressed each of the strategy steps. If you missed any steps, follow up with the implementer. It is important to make sure that the strategies were delivered as planned so that they have the most likelihood of impacting the implementer. If there were any adaptations made to the intervention plan during action planning, *update the intervention plan.* Next, *complete the Summary Report for Implementation Planning* (Appendix 5.4) to document the logistics as well as the strategies to address anticipated barriers identified during implementation planning. Share the updated materials with the implementer as soon as possible. *Obtain any resources for which you are responsible* according to the Action Plan Worksheet, Part B (Appendix 5.2B) and give them to the implementer as soon as possible. Last, *check in with the implementer following the meeting to touch base about intervention fidelity and answer his or her questions.* This follow-up will ensure that the implementer

---

BOX 5.4. Follow-Up Steps after Implementation Planning

1. Review session notes to ensure that the strategy was delivered as planned.
2. Update intervention plan, as needed.
3. Complete the Summary Report for Implementation Planning (Appendix 5.4).
4. Obtain any resources for which you are responsible.
5. Check in with the implementer following the meeting to touch base about intervention fidelity and answer his or her questions.

feels comfortable delivering the intervention after the meeting and that his or her questions have been answered. Confirm that the implementer knows how to contact you with any questions about the intervention or its implementation.

SUMMARY

Implementation planning prepares the implementer to deliver an intervention by outlining, in detail, the logistics of each individual step of the intervention as well as by identifying barriers to implementation and strategies to overcome those barriers. It was developed to act as a link between intending to and engaging in a new behavior (in this case, intervention implementation), based on a theory in health psychology, and has been documented as effective with varied implementers responsible for individualized, targeted, and group interventions. To support the implementer, we recommend that this strategy be implemented, alone or in conjunction with direct training, before the intervention is implemented. It can also be updated if intervention fidelity is low during the delivery of the intervention. At the conclusion of the implementation planning session, the implementer will be ready to deliver the intervention, which has been adapted to his or her context and clearly delineated, with high levels of intervention fidelity.

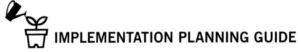

APPENDIX 5.1
Implementation Planning Guide

Consultant: _____   Implementer: _____   Date: _____

Learner: _____   Intervention: _____   Start/End Time: _____

🌱 READINESS CHECKLIST

✓	Have you . . .
1. Reviewed the intervention and current data?	
☐	Familiarized yourself with and broken down the intervention plan?
	If using implementation planning after implementation has already begun:
☐	Reviewed the intervention goal and, using data, the learner's current progress?
☐	Evaluated intervention fidelity data?
2. Prepared for implementation planning?	
☐	Read about implementation planning?
☐	Prepared Action and Coping Plan Worksheets (Appendix 5.2A–5.2E)?
☐	Practiced dialogue, as needed, to be comfortable at the meeting?
3. Identified session logistics?	
☐	Scheduled the implementation planning session?
☐	Reached out to the implementer?
☐	Brought implementation planning materials to the session?

🪴 IMPLEMENTATION PLANNING GUIDE

Step 1: Explain the Purpose of the Session

- Provide an overview of implementation planning.
- Begin implementation planning in an open, supportive manner.

Following is an example of what you might say to explain the purpose of this session.

> "Today, we're here to talk about the intervention and develop an implementation plan. Completion of an implementation plan is a three-step process. First we will review background information about the selected intervention and the recipient(s). Second, we will break down the intervention into smaller, more specific steps, and then complete action planning regarding the details

(continued)

of implementation. Third, we will complete coping planning to problem-solve any barriers to implementation. This planning process is designed to facilitate the definition and adaptation of the intervention so that it fits your specific intervention context/classroom."

_____

_____

_____

Step 2: Review the Target Concern and Goal

- Review the target concern, current data, and intervention goal.
- Describe generally how the intervention can address the learner's issue and support the learner to meet his or her goal.

  "Just to orient us, you referred [*student*]/sought my consultation about [*group/classroom*] due to your concerns about [*behavior(s) of concern*]. [*Intervention*] was selected because when implemented well, it will help [*learner*] meet his or her goal. We will review and refine [*intervention*] to fit your context/classroom today."

_____

_____

_____

Step 3: Review Intervention Steps

- Show the implementer the list of intervention steps (on Action Plan Worksheet: Part A).
- Discuss if the organization of intervention steps makes sense; if not, revise.

  "[*Show Action Plan Worksheet, Part A*] To begin, let's review the steps for carrying out this intervention for [*learner*]. As you can see, I have filled in the intervention steps in the first two columns of the worksheet. It is important to make sure that we to include all components of the intervention when describing the intervention steps."

_____

_____

_____

Step 4: Modify the Intervention Steps, If Needed

- Ask the implementer if modifications to intervention steps could increase feasibility or contextual fit.
- Keep in mind the empirical and theoretical support for any modifications to intervention steps.

  "Before we get into planning the logistics of implementation, let's first look at each intervention step to see if there are any potential revisions that we need to discuss. Please read through these intervention steps again and let me know if there are any steps that you would like to discuss."

  (continued)

[Write revisions beside the corresponding intervention step in the third column of the Action Plan Worksheet, Part A.]

_____

_____

_____

Step 5: Identify the Logistics of Each Intervention Step

- Discuss how proactively planning logistics of an intervention can help implementation.
- Ask the implementer to identify logistics of the implementation and any needed resources.
- Record implementer responses regarding intervention logistics on Action Plan Worksheet, Part B.

  "Thinking about the specific details for each intervention step helps ensure that we are on the same page regarding implementation and that you are confident in what you need to do and how it will fit in your context. The first intervention step is [*state the step*]. When will you implement this step? . . . How often will you implement this step? . . . For how long will you implement this step? . . . Where will you implement this step? . . . Do you need any additional resources to implement this step?"

_____

_____

_____

Step 6: Discuss How Needed Resources May Be Obtained, if Applicable

- Identify how, when, and by whom the needed resources can be obtained.
- Record plan for obtaining resources on Action Plan Worksheet, Part C

  "We identified a few additional materials that are needed to fully implement this intervention plan. For example, you need a self-monitoring form for the student. I can develop this form and email it to you by the end of the week. You also need more books that are at the student's reading level. Can you work with the reading specialist to obtain these by the end of this week as well?"

_____

_____

_____

Step 7: Summarize the Action Plan

- Summarize revisions made (if applicable) and the logistical details of implementation.
- Praise the implementer for his or her participation in the process.

  "Great, thanks for your excellent input regarding how you will be able to implement this intervention. We made a few revisions [*if applicable*] such as [*name revisions*] to better align the intervention with your routines. Then you determined the specific logistics of how each

(continued)

intervention step will be implemented in your classroom/context. Finally, you identified a few items that we need to obtain for you to be able to best implement the intervention."

Step 8: Identify Potential Barriers to Implementation

- Ask the implementer to identify major anticipated or current barriers to intervention implementation.
- Ask the implementer to prioritize his or her top four barriers.
- Record barriers on Coping Plan Worksheet.

"Even with the best planning, there may be barriers that could interfere with your plans to implement an intervention. The purpose of completing a Coping Plan Worksheet is to proactively identify a few potential major barriers to intervention implementation and to develop strategies to deal with those barriers. In this way, if barriers arise, they should be easier to overcome so that implementation is maintained. What barriers do you anticipate/are you experiencing that might/will affect your implementation of this intervention? How would you rank the priority of each barrier as compared to the others?"

Step 9: Identify Potential Strategies to Address Barriers

- Brainstorm ways to maintain implementation in presence of each barrier.
- Write identified strategies on Coping Plan Worksheet.

"Great job thinking of some barriers that might hinder your implementation. Let's review each of the top four and think about how you might be able to maintain implementation of the intervention if/when you encounter the barrier. So for the first barrier [*state barrier*], what do you think you could do? What do you think about [*provide suggestion*]?"

(continued)

Step 10: Summarize Coping Planning

- Summarize the strategies identified to address barriers.
- Praise the implementer for his or her participation in the process.

> "Thanks for brainstorming strategies to ameliorate the major barriers. These strategies should give you confidence to address these barriers if or when they arise during implementation."

_____

_____

_____

Step 11: Review the Meeting and Thank the Implementer

- Review the meeting discussion and decisions.
- Thank the implementer and close the meeting.

> "We made a few revisions to the plan, such as [*provide example of a revision*]. We also determined the specifics of how the intervention will be implemented in your classroom. I am responsible for getting [*name resources*] to you by [*day/time*]. You are going to get [*name resources*]. You also identified a few barriers you anticipate might come up, and we brainstormed a few ideas of how you can handle these barriers should they arise. Do you have any questions about what we've covered? I will provide you with a clean copy of the implementation plan by [*day/time*]. What would be a good day and time for us to meet or check in again? Thank you for taking the time to discuss this intervention plan."

_____

_____

_____

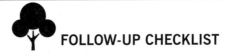 **FOLLOW-UP CHECKLIST**

✓	Have you . . .
☐	1. Reviewed session notes to ensure that the strategy was delivered as planned?
☐	2. Updated the intervention plan, as needed?
☐	3. Completed the Summary Report for Implementation Planning?
☐	4. Obtained any resources for which you were responsible?
☐	5. Checked in with the implementer following the meeting to touch base about intervention fidelity and answered his or her questions?

Action Plan Worksheet

Intervention Step #	Intervention Step	Revision to Intervention Step (if applicable)

Action Plan Worksheet

Intervention Step #	To Be Implemented				Resources Needed?
	When?	How Often?	For How Long?	Where?	

Action Plan Worksheet

Intervention Step #	Resources Needed		
	What?	Who Is Responsible?	By When?

Action Plan Sample Responses

When?		
☐ Gen Ed—homeroom	☐ Special education— inclusion	☐ During bus ride
☐ Gen Ed—reading/language arts/English	☐ Special education—resource room	☐ During assemblies
☐ Gen Ed—math		☐ Before school
☐ Gen Ed—science	☐ Teacher aide present	☐ After school
☐ Gen Ed—social studies/ history	☐ Special education aide present	☐ During prep period
☐ Gen Ed—foreign language	☐ During lunch	☐ When teacher with the student(s)
☐ Gen Ed—other	☐ Before school	☐ All day
☐ Music	☐ After school	☐ All morning
☐ Physical education	☐ During recess	☐ All afternoon
☐ Technology	☐ In place of instruction time (specify)	☐ When student exhibits _____ behavior/skill (specify)
☐ Chorus	☐ During study hall/free period	☐ When student doesn't exhibit _____ behavior/skill
☐ Orchestra	☐ During transitions	
☐ Band		

How often?		
☐ Once	☐ Hourly	☐ _____ weeks/month
☐ Every _____ minutes	☐ _____ times/day	☐ Monthly
☐ _____ times/period	☐ Daily	☐ _____ days/marking period
☐ _____ times/activity	☐ _____ days/week	☐ _____ weeks/marking period
☐ At the beginning of _____	☐ Weekly	☐ As needed
☐ At the end of _____	☐ _____ days/month	☐ Other (specify)

For how long?		
☐ Throughout _____ instruction (specify)	☐ For _____ minutes (specify)	☐ Other (specify)
☐ Throughout period	☐ As long as needed	☐ Until step completed
	☐ Throughout activity	☐ Not applicable

(continued)

Where? General locations

- ☐ Gen Ed classroom—homeroom
- ☐ Gen Ed classroom—reading/ELA/English
- ☐ Gen Ed classroom—math
- ☐ Gen Ed classroom—science
- ☐ Gen Ed classroom—social studies/history
- ☐ Gen Ed classroom—foreign language
- ☐ Gen Ed classroom—when class not in session
- ☐ Gen Ed classroom—other (specify)
- ☐ Special education—resource room
- ☐ Special education—resource room—when class not in session
- ☐ Music classroom
- ☐ Technology classroom
- ☐ Chorus classroom
- ☐ Cafeteria
- ☐ General purpose room
- ☐ Theatre
- ☐ Band
- ☐ Library
- ☐ Bathroom
- ☐ Hallway
- ☐ School office
- ☐ School psychologist's office
- ☐ School counselor's office
- ☐ School social worker's office

- ☐ Gym
- ☐ Playground
- ☐ Bus
- ☐ Empty classroom
- ☐ Empty conference room
- ☐ Empty office
- ☐ Home
- ☐ Other (specify)
- ☐ At teacher's desk
- ☐ At student's desk
- ☐ At station(s)/center(s)
- ☐ At table
- ☐ At/near cubbies
- ☐ At lab table
- ☐ Wherever the student is
- ☐ At computer
- ☐ On rug
- ☐ On floor
- ☐ In girls' bathroom—at sinks
- ☐ In boys' bathroom—at sinks
- ☐ In girls' bathroom—in stalls
- ☐ In boys' bathroom—in stalls
- ☐ In boys' bathroom—at urinal
- ☐ At/on chalk/whiteboard
- ☐ In locker room
- ☐ On stage
- ☐ On field
- ☐ On track
- ☐ In library stacks

- ☐ Immediately outside classroom
- ☐ In hallway leading to next class/activity
- ☐ In study hall
- ☐ In principal's office
- ☐ In vice principal's office
- ☐ Near administrative assistant's desk
- ☐ In nurse's office
- ☐ In chair/seat
- ☐ On play equipment
- ☐ On playground
- ☐ In bedroom
- ☐ In living room
- ☐ In kitchen
- ☐ In dining room
- ☐ In parents' bedroom
- ☐ In sibling's bedroom
- ☐ In backyard
- ☐ In front yard
- ☐ In side yard
- ☐ Other (specify)

Coping Plan Worksheet

Priority	Barrier to Intervention Implementation	Strategy to Continue Implementation

Fidelity Data Sheet for Implementation Planning

For each of the strategy steps, provide a rating of adherence (to what extent you covered each step) and of quality (how well you delivered each step) based on the following rubric.

Adherence	Quality
2 = All components of the step delivered. 1 = Some components of the step delivered. 0 = No components of the step delivered.	2 = Step delivered in a smooth, natural manner, responsive to the implementer, and with appropriate nonverbal interaction. 1 = Step delivered with some aspects of quality. 0 = Step delivered without any aspects of quality.

Strategy Steps	Adherence	Quality
1. Explain purpose of session.		
2. Review the target concern and goal.		
3. Review the intervention steps.		
4. Modify the intervention steps, if needed.		
5. Identify the logistics of each intervention step.		
6. Discuss how needed resources may be obtained, if applicable.		
7. Summarize the action plan.		
8. Identify potential barriers to implementation.		
9. Identify potential strategies to address any barriers.		
10. Summarize the coping planning.		
11. Thank the implementer for meeting.		

First, sum each column: _____   _____

22   22

Next, divide by number of steps to identify a percentage: = _____%   = _____%

Summary Report for Implementation Planning

Intervention Recipient: _____   Implementer: _____

Date Written: _____   Consultant: _____

This implementation plan is based on collaborative decisions concerning how implementation of the intervention can best fit within the context of the current classroom and potential barriers to implementation in this context. The purpose of this action plan portion is to document the intervention implementation steps and the detailed logistical planning regarding how each step will be implemented. The purpose of the coping plan portion is to identify barriers to initiating and sustaining implementation and to develop a plan to maintain implementation when barriers are encountered. The first section outlines the action plan for each intervention step and the second section outlines potential barriers and strategies to maintain implementation.

I. Action Plan

Intervention Step	To Be Implemented				Resources Needed?
	When?	How Often?	For How Long?	Where?	

(continued)

Summary Report for Implementation Planning *(page 2 of 3)*

Intervention Step	To Be Implemented				Resources Needed?
	When?	How Often?	For How Long?	Where?	

(continued)

Summary Report for Implementation Planning *(page 3 of 3)*

Intervention Step	To Be Implemented				Resources Needed?
	When?	How Often?	For How Long?	Where?	

II. Coping Plan

Potential Major Barrier to Intervention Implementation	Strategy to Implement the Intervention Nevertheless

Note. If the intervention is modified (e.g., new components added or removed, implemented in new context) or new barriers are identified during implementation, the Action and Coping Plan Worksheets may be updated as needed.

CHAPTER 6

Direct Training

WHAT IS DIRECT TRAINING?

The overall purpose of direct training is to prepare the implementer to deliver the intervention with fidelity by teaching him or her foundational intervention knowledge and skills (Box 6.1). During direct training, you will provide didactic training on intervention steps, demonstrate the intervention, give the implementer the opportunity to practice the intervention first with guidance and then independently, and provide positive yet corrective feedback. After direct training, the implementer will have an increased understanding of

---

BOX 6.1. Direct Training Snapshot

Who?	Implementers who are new to an intervention (i.e., before intervention implementation) or who do not understand how to deliver some or all of the intervention steps during the course of intervention implementation.
What?	An introduction to how and why each intervention step is delivered, a demonstration of the intervention, and the opportunity for guided and then independent practice for the implementer with ongoing feedback.
Where? When?	Deliver it during a one-time session in a private meeting space.
Why?	It includes (1) a detailed description of the intervention and how it is delivered, (2) modeling to illustrate intervention fidelity, and (3) the opportunity to practice with feedback until mastery is achieved.

---

the intervention, a positive experience of delivering the intervention steps, and more optimistic expectations about intervention effectiveness and the feasibility of delivering the intervention with fidelity.

It is likely that you have provided aspects of direct training in your previous efforts to support implementers, in that components of direct training are often included in professional development, consultation, and coaching activities (e.g., Joyce & Showers, 2002; Kratochwill et al., 2014). Although it is possible that these efforts have been helpful for some implementers, comprehensive direct training (i.e., didactic instruction, modeling, practice, and feedback) has been shown to be more effective than other types of training in increasing implementers' intervention fidelity (e.g., Sterling-Turner, Watson, Wildmon, Watkins, & Little, 2001; Sterling-Turner et al., 2002). Direct training can include modeling via video (Bice-Urbach & Kratochwill, 2016; DiGennaro Reed, Codding, Catania, & Maguire, 2010), and it has been documented as an effective implementation support for implementers who are delivering academic and behavioral interventions (e.g., Dib & Sturmey, 2007; Fallon, Sanetti, et al., 2018; Sterling-Turner et al., 2002).

RESEARCH ON DIRECT TRAINING

Direct training has been evaluated in the research literature as an independent implementation support (e.g., Fallon, Sanetti, et al., 2018; Sterling-Turner et al., 2001, 2002) and as a component of consultation and coaching (Joyce & Showers, 2002; Kratochwill et al., 2014). It has been consistently demonstrated to be an effective, proactive strategy that can increase the intervention fidelity of teachers (Dufrene et al., 2012; Sarakoff & Sturmey, 2004) and parents (Miles & Wilder, 2009) implementing academic (Fallon, Sanetti, et al., 2018) and behavioral (Sterling-Turner et al., 2002) interventions. A recent systematic review of single-case-design studies documented strong effect sizes associated with the application of direct training on adults' behavior in school settings (Fallon, Kurtz, & Mueller, 2018). Although, in some cases, direct training alone has been found to be unable to sustain a high level of intervention fidelity, it can be effective in the long term for some implementers (Sanetti & Collier-Meek, 2015). Further, direct training is an efficient way to initially introduce an implementer to an intervention and teach him or her how to deliver it with fidelity.

HOW DOES DIRECT TRAINING WORK?

Direct training can be explained in terms of behavioral theory (Cooper et al., 2007) and social learning theory (Bandura, 1977). Behavioral theory suggests that individuals learn new behaviors by engaging in those behaviors and directly experiencing their consequences (i.e., operant conditioning; Cooper et al., 2007). During direct training, the implementer is given an opportunity to practice the intervention in a supportive environment and to receive positive yet corrective feedback until mastery is achieved (Jenkins & DiGennaro Reed, 2016). In this way, the implementer learns the new intervention through actually engaging the new behavior and receiving positive reinforcement. Social learning theory incorporates behavioral and cognitive frameworks and describes observational learning and imitation to be a foundational way to learn new behaviors (Bandura, 1977). That is, we learn by observing models, considering the consequences of these behaviors modeled, and deciding to enact these behaviors ourselves. To learn a new behavior through modeling, social learning theory suggests that implementers must (1) attend to the modeled behavior, (2) remember the behavior, (3) be able to reproduce the behavior, and (4) be motivated to do so (Bandura, 1977). As such, when delivering direct training, it may be helpful to ensure that these conditions are met as you support the implementer to learn the intervention.

WHAT IMPLEMENTERS WILL BENEFIT FROM DIRECT TRAINING?

We recommend that direct training be delivered before intervention delivery begins, but it can also be provided during intervention implementation if an implementer is struggling to deliver an intervention with adequate fidelity. When provided before intervention implementation begins, direct training prepares the implementer by providing a detailed introduction to the intervention and opportunity to practice delivering it successfully before actually being in the target environment with the learner. It can also be an opportunity to proactively address any questions or concerns the implementer might have about the intervention. As such, direct training is particularly important when an implementer has never provided a similar intervention, the intervention is complex, or the outcome is a high-stakes one (e.g., lack of responsiveness may result in outplacement). However, we have found that it can be a helpful strategy to deliver direct training even to veteran implementers to prompt them to the rationale for intervention and specific aspects of intervention fidelity (e.g., provide examples of quality delivery, remind them about exposure). We suggest that direct training be delivered in conjunction with implementation planning so that you and the implementer first planfully adapt the intervention to the implementation context and then provide direct training on the adapted intervention; however, it can also be delivered as a stand-alone implementation support. When provided during intervention implementation, direct training is well suited to address skill-based deficits (i.e., low levels of intervention fidelity due to a lack skill) because of its focus on modeling and practice. At this point, direct training can involve a review of the whole intervention, or it can target the intervention steps that the implementer is not delivering consistently. Direct training is the least resource-intensive of the skill-building implementation supports (see Chapter 3).

GETTING READY FOR DIRECT TRAINING

Direct training involves intervention review, modeling, and practice that can incorporate intervention fidelity data, if it is available (i.e., during intervention implementation). As such, the preparation required depends on when direct training is delivered in the implementation process. Overall, getting ready to deliver direct training involves three steps, outlined in Box 6.2 and described in the following sections.

BOX 6.2. Getting Ready to Deliver Direct Training

1. Review the intervention and current data.
   - Familiarize yourself with the intervention plan.
   - Review the intervention goal and, using data, the learner's current progress.
   - Review intervention fidelity data, if available.

2. Prepare for direct training.
   - Read about direct training.
   - Practice dialogue, as needed, to be comfortable at the meeting.

3. Identify session logistics.
   - Schedule direct training session.
   - Reach out to the implementer.
   - Bring direct training materials to the session.

Step 1: Review the Intervention and Current Data

To prepare for direct training, *familiarize yourself with the intervention plan* so that you are able to fluently describe the how-to and the why of each intervention step as well as model and support the implementer to deliver these steps with intervention fidelity. During the meeting, the implementer will refer to your expertise on delivering the intervention with fidelity; be prepared to serve in this role. If not already completed, break down the intervention into components. To do so, consider how the intervention plan might be best taught to the implementer. Divide the intervention plan into grouped intervention steps that will help the implementer understand (1) the overall intervention plan and (2) how the intervention steps fit into the larger components of the intervention. For example, you could group intervention steps according to *when* the steps must be implemented (e.g., all steps delivered at once, different steps provided at separate times) or in relation to the theoretical links between the intervention steps (e.g., if several steps are based on one principle, if intervention steps build on one another). If available, *review the intervention goal and learner's progress,* and *review intervention fidelity data.* Knowing the specifics of the learner's goals and current progress will help you effectively convey how the intervention is designed to impact the learner. If intervention fidelity data are available, the information can be used in training, modeling, and practice to focus on the intervention steps that the implementer is not delivering consistently. For instance, if an implementer demonstrates low adherence and quality when delivering a particular step, you should emphasize this step during direct training (e.g., review aspects of the intervention step that have been missed, reference specific aspects of the intervention step during modeling, be very positive about improvements to these intervention steps during practice).

Step 2: Prepare for Direct Training

To be comfortable delivering this strategy, carefully *read about direct training* to familiarize yourself with the strategy steps and talking points. Confirm your understanding of
the purpose of the strategy and each of the steps. Prepare any necessary information or
materials (e.g., written intervention plan, research). To *practice your dialogue,* read the
Direct Training Guide (see Appendix 6.1) and, if available, review intervention fidelity data
and learner outcome data. This preparation will help you to maximize the strategy session
and feel comfortable addressing the implementer's concerns and needs. As noted above, it
may be helpful to (1) organize the intervention into a written list of teachable steps for the
purpose of demonstration and practice, (2) identify target steps for practice based on implementation data, and/or (3) brainstorm potential scenarios to use for practicing target steps.

Step 3: Identify Session Logistics

Once ready, it is necessary to plan the session logistics. To *schedule direct training,* determine how long the meeting will last, when to hold the meeting, how many sessions are
needed to complete the strategy, and whether to use technology to facilitate the meeting.
Plan to meet for approximately 30 minutes, although some direct training sessions may be
shorter or longer, depending on the intervention and the implementer's skill. Decide who
will be involved (e.g., primary implementer, potential collaborators). In some cases, there
is more than one person implementing the intervention (e.g., paraprofessionals, school support professionals), or other stakeholders (e.g., case worker, parent), who may be interested
in attending. Arrange where you will meet. You will need a quiet space that offers privacy
for modeling and practice. Make sure that the time and location are feasible for the implementer. You may decide to deliver modeling via video in some cases (e.g., many people need
to get trained on this intervention, the implementer might want to view a model regularly).
If using video, consider the logistics of shooting the video, including accessing the necessary technology, making time to model the intervention, and having someone videotape you
and edit the product, if needed. *Reach out to the implementer* ahead of the direct training
session. If you think it would be helpful for the implementer to review any materials prior
to the strategy meeting, provide those in advance (e.g., written list of intervention steps,
sample intervention materials, research, data). *Bring direct training materials* to the session, including the Direct Training Guide (Appendix 6.1), the written intervention plan,
and, if available, graphs of intervention fidelity and learner outcome data.

DIRECT TRAINING STEP-BY-STEP

Direct training involves didactic training on intervention steps; demonstration of the intervention; and implementer practice with positive yet corrective feedback, first with guidance
and then independently. The six steps of a typical direct training session are listed in Box
6.3. These steps remain the same whether direct training is delivered in person or partially

---

BOX 6.3. Direct Training Steps

1. Explain the purpose of the session.
2. Provide didactic intervention training.
3. Demonstrate the intervention.
4. Engage the implementer in guided practice.
5. Engage the implementer in independent practice.
6. Review the meeting and thank the implementer.

---

or fully delivered via video. The Direct Training Guide at the end of this chapter includes the steps, key objectives, and sample language, as well as space for recording an implementer's responses. This guide can be copied and used for delivering this implementation support in your practice. A description of the steps involved in direct training, including key objectives and quick tips for delivery, are provided in the following sections.

Step 1: Explain the Purpose of the Session

- Provide an overview of direct training.
- Begin direct training in an open, supportive manner.

As direct training begins, provide an overview to help the implementer understand how the session will unfold and what his or her role will be. Explain that you will be reviewing the intervention plan, demonstrating the intervention steps, providing an opportunity for the implementer to practice the intervention steps, and giving feedback to ensure the he or she masters the intervention. Consider asking the implementer if there are any additional items he or she would like to add to the agenda. This approach can help set a tone of collaboration and active engagement during the session.

Step 2: Provide Didactic Intervention Training

- Describe the how and why of each intervention step.
- Elicit and answer the implementer's questions about the intervention.

Provide didactic training to ensure that the implementer understands the purpose of and how to implement each intervention step. To do so, review each intervention step. Provide detailed instructions about how to carry out each step, making sure to address the attributes of adherence, quality, and exposure, as applicable. If the implementer is not introduced to an aspect of the intervention, he or she won't know to incorporate it into his or her intervention delivery. As such, it's critical to be comprehensive in your description of the intervention. As you review each step, emphasize *why* each intervention step is important and *what* it is designed to accomplish by describing relevant theory and research. Make the link between the intervention steps and the effectiveness of the intervention for the particular

Quick Tip 6.1. Encouraging the Implementer's Questions

 Ask the implementer questions to elicit his or her opinions, concerns, or questions about the intervention. Go beyond generic questions that simply require a yes or no answer, such as "Do you have any questions?" or "Does that make sense?." Instead, have the implementer consider his or her impressions of the intervention, how the intervention will fit into classroom routines, and what potential questions or issues may arise during implementation. Following is a list of potential questions to include during direct training and your other consultation meetings. Use these and similar questions to guide your consultation.

- "How do you see that intervention step happening in your classroom?"
- "Have you delivered interventions like this one in the past? Tell me about your experience."
- "What do you think will be easiest about delivering this intervention? Which intervention steps might be challenging?"
- "To which intervention steps do you see the student being particularly responsive?"
- "How will you describe this intervention to the student's parents?"

It is OK to ask the implementer in return what he or she might think about his or her own question or concern (e.g., "In your experience, how have you handled that issue?"). Inherent in this consultation process is a valuing of both your skills and knowledge *and* those of the implementer. The types of responses emphasized here will reinforce the collaboration and mutual trust that are critical to your relationship with the implementer.

learner. Helping the implementer to understand the rationale of the intervention steps can reinforce the importance of delivering the intervention with fidelity. Providing the implementer with a written copy of the intervention plan can help facilitate didactic training by allowing the implementer to follow along with your explanations of each step and by providing a place to take notes.

Throughout your review of the intervention, ask the implementer to share his or her questions to facilitate a supportive and interactive dialogue. It is likely the implementer will have questions about the rationale for specific steps or how to deliver the intervention with fidelity. Address the implementer's questions and concerns as best you can, based on intervention-related research and your experience. It is important to validate the thoughtfulness and perspective of the implementer's questions and concerns (e.g., "Great question! I had not thought of that"; "I see why you might have a concern about that step. In my experience . . ."). At the end of this didactic instruction, the implementer should understand why each intervention steps is necessary and how it is designed to impact learner outcomes, as well as the basics of how to deliver the intervention with fidelity. The implementer should also feel that his or her general questions have been welcomed and answered.

Step 3: Demonstrate the Intervention

- Model how to deliver the intervention with fidelity.

Next, demonstrate the intervention to provide a model of how to deliver each step of it. In most cases, the modeling will occur in person, during the meeting, but if you decided to use video modeling, refer to Quick Tip 6.2 on page 109 for suggestions. Depending on the intervention, it may be helpful for the implementer to act as the learner. Initially, you may be hesitant or uncomfortable about engaging in this process with your colleague, the implementer; however, research strongly supports the benefits of this approach (Sterling-Turner et al., 2001, 2002). Further, it is possible to make this process feel natural and supportive. To model the intervention, (1) provide examples of how you might deliver particular steps or (2) explain how you might respond to particular scenarios by implementing the intervention (e.g., "If Johnny calls out, I would respond by . . ."). While modeling, describe what you are doing to implement the intervention, linking this description to your review of the intervention steps earlier. Use intervention materials, as appropriate.

During the demonstration, make sure to attend to the dimensions of adherence, exposure, and quality. Make sure your demonstration of the intervention matches your description of the intervention steps you provided during the didactic training portion (adherence). To address exposure, indicate how long certain intervention steps should take, especially if your demonstration is just a snapshot (e.g., "Now I would walk around the room like this while the learners work independently for 10 minutes"). To address quality, indicate (as appropriate) the (1) important aspects of your interaction with the learner (e.g., tone of voice, nonverbal behaviors; "When I prompt the learner, I will use a neutral, calm tone of voice"); (2) fluency of your intervention delivery (e.g., responding to a student immediately, having materials readily accessible); (3) the timing of your behaviors (e.g., "Notice how I provided clear, concise three-step instructions before beginning the activity"); and (4) responsive aspects of your delivery (e.g., "When I saw that the learner was skipping lines in her repeated reading, I gave her a bookmark to place under the line she is reading").

Step 4: Engage the Implementer in Guided Practice

- Have the implementer practice the intervention with your active support.
- Provide positive yet corrective feedback.
- Repeat guided practice until the implementer is ready to practice delivering the intervention independently

Guided practice gives the implementer an opportunity to practice the new skills needed to deliver the intervention in a supportive environment. In direct training, this *guided* practice occurs before *independent* practice (Step 5). Guided practice allows for more supported, collaborative rehearsal of the intervention steps with you, whereas independent practice allows the implementer to demonstrate that he or she can deliver each intervention step without your support. To engage the implementer in guided practice, ask him or her to practice the intervention and provide supportive guidance as needed. To start the implementer's practice, it may be helpful to offer a scenario, ask him or her to pick an intervention step, or simply begin at the beginning of the intervention (if it's sequential in nature). You can provide the implementer with guidance in the form of additional explanations of intervention steps, prompts, hints, guiding questions, answering the implementer's questions, and encouragement. You can provide such guidance by stopping the practice outright to discuss something or by providing small suggestions while practice is underway. Give the implementer the materials with which to implement each intervention step, as necessary.

Quick Tip 6.2. Strategies to Make Demonstration and Practice Comfortable for Implementers

Some implementers may be a bit uncomfortable with the demonstration and practice components, so take care to make sure that the process is as comfortable and naturalistic as possible. To do so, set up your demonstration as an opportunity to share examples and use scenarios from the implementer's setting that you have observed (e.g., "To deliver this step, at the beginning of circle time you might say . . ." or "When you're handing out papers would be a great time for you to . . ."). After providing the demonstration, ask a question to facilitate the practice (e.g., "So, that's how it could look at circle time. What might you say during independent seatwork?"; "So, in your own words, what do you think you'll plan to say when you're handing out papers?"). In this way, the demonstration and practice remain a natural part of the conversation around implementation.

Following the guided practice, provide feedback to the implementer about his or her intervention fidelity. In your feedback, be specific as you refer to each intervention step in a positive and constructive manner. Be sure to reinforce successes and correct any intervention fidelity errors. Share with the implementer the particular steps he or she implemented according to plan and/or with sufficient quality and exposure, and the steps on which he or she should focus to improve his or her adherence, quality, or exposure. The implementer should feel more confident and positive about delivering the intervention following appropriate and reinforcing feedback.

Some implementers will benefit from repeated guided practice and feedback. Ask the implementer about his or her knowledge of and confidence in delivering the intervention. If it appears the implementer needs more guided practice to feel confident delivering the intervention, repeat guided practice until the he or she successfully delivers the intervention with fidelity. Subsequent rounds of guided practice do not have to be identical to the initial practice. Consider fading the intensity of guidance to help the implementer transition successfully from guided to independent practice.

Step 5: Engage the Implementer in Independent Practice

- Have the implementer practice the intervention independently.
- Provide positive yet corrective feedback.
- Repeat independent practice until the implementer is prepared to deliver the intervention with fluency and fidelity.

During independent practice, the implementer will deliver the intervention without guidance. This independent practice will give the implementer an additional opportunity to ensure that he or she is prepared and confident to deliver the intervention with fidelity. To engage the implementer in independent practice, ask him or her to independently practice the intervention or grouped intervention steps, either from the first step or in response to a scenario. Do not provide any guidance during the independent practice, but take note of areas of strength as well as areas for improvement. In doing so, identify the implementer's level of adherence, quality, and exposure.

After the independent practice, ask the implementer to reflect on his or her performance. In doing so, help the implementer identify which steps he or she delivered with sufficient intervention fidelity, and which steps still need improvement. The self-evaluation might also result in additional questions or concerns about the intervention plan. Provide constructive feedback regarding the implementer's independent practice. Remember to keep feedback positive and constructive. In doing so, be sure to correct any implementation errors, but also reinforce successes.

As with the guided practice, examine the implementer's skill and confidence during the independent practice and his or her response to feedback. If the implementer needs more practice to confidently deliver the intervention with adequate fidelity, repeat the practice. Provide additional independent practice and feedback until the implementer successfully delivers each component of the intervention without your support.

Step 6: Review the Meeting and Thank the Implementer

- Review the meeting discussion and decisions.
- Thank the implementer and close the meeting.

The implementer should leave the direct training session with a solid understanding of the intervention and confidence in his or her ability to deliver it with fidelity. Review the meeting and provide positive feedback to the implementer about his or her participation and growth. Highlight the link between the intervention steps, intervention fidelity, and changes in outcomes for the learner. Before closing the session, ask the implementer if he or she has any remaining questions about delivering the intervention plan. End the meeting by thanking the implementer for engaging with you during direct training and encouraging him or her to be in touch with you if intervention fidelity issues arise.

FOLLOW-UP AFTER DIRECT TRAINING

To solidify the discussion and practice that occurred during direct training, we suggest that you engage in some activities after the session. Follow-up after direct training involves three steps, outlined in Box 6.4 and described below.

Review session notes to ensure that the strategy was delivered as planned. To do so, check the Direct Training Guide (Appendix 6.1) and complete a self-assessment using the Fidelity Data Sheet for Direct Training (Appendix 6.2) to see if you addressed each of the

---

BOX 6.4. Follow-Up Steps after Direct Training

1. Review session notes to ensure that the strategy was delivered as planned.
2. Update the intervention plan and/or implementation plan, as needed.
3. Check in with the implementer following the meeting to touch base about intervention fidelity and answer his or her questions.

strategy steps. If you missed any steps, follow up with the implementer. It is important to make sure that the strategies were delivered as planned so that they have the most likelihood of impacting the implementer. If needed, *update the intervention plan and/or the implementation plan.* If any changes were made during direct training, update these written materials to reflect those changes. Share the updated materials with the implementer as soon as possible. Last, *check in with implementer following the meeting to touch base about intervention fidelity and answer his or her questions.* This follow-up will ensure that the implementer feels comfortable delivering the intervention after the meeting and that his or her questions have been answered. Confirm that the implementer knows how to contact you with any questions about the intervention or its implementation.

SUMMARY

Direct training prepares implementers to deliver interventions with high levels of fidelity by teaching foundational intervention knowledge and skills, including didactic training on intervention steps, demonstration of the intervention, the opportunity for the implementer to practice the intervention first with guidance and then independently, and the delivery of positive and targeted feedback. We recommend that you provide direct training in conjunction with implementation planning (Chapter 5) prior to any implementation, although it can also be delivered alone. If low levels of intervention fidelity are documented, direct training can be provided to address skill-based deficits. After direct training, the implementer will better understand and have a positive experience with delivering the intervention steps with fidelity.

APPENDIX 6.1
Direct Training Guide

Consultant: _____   Implementer: _____   Date: _____

Learner: _____   Intervention: _____   Start/End Time: _____

READINESS CHECKLIST

✓	Have you . . .
	1. Reviewed the intervention and current data?
☐	Familiarized yourself with the intervention plan?
☐	Reviewed the intervention goal and learner's current progress?
☐	Reviewed intervention fidelity data?
	2. Prepared for direct training?
☐	Read about direct training?
☐	Practiced dialogue, as needed, to be comfortable at the meeting?
	3. Identified session logistics?
☐	Scheduled direct training?
☐	Reached out to the implementer?
☐	Brought direct training materials to the session?

DIRECT TRAINING GUIDE

Step 1: Explain the Purpose of the Session

- Provide an overview of direct training.
- Begin direct training in an open, supportive manner.

Following is an example of what you might say to explain the purpose of this session.

> "Today, we're here to talk about the [*intervention*]. We'll go through the steps in detail and have time for some practice together. By the end of our meeting, you should feel confident about delivering the intervention."

_____

_____

_____

_____

(continued)

Step 2: Provide Didactic Intervention Training

- Describe the how and why of each intervention step.
- Elicit and answer the implementer's questions about the intervention.

"Let's start with the first step. To deliver it you will [*describe how to deliver intervention step*], which is important because it [*describe why the intervention step matters*]."

_____

_____

_____

_____

_____

Step 3: Demonstrate the Intervention

- Model how to deliver the intervention with fidelity.

"So, when starting the intervention, you might say [*demonstrate intervention*]. If [*learner*] responds inappropriately, you would [*demonstrate intervention*]."

_____

_____

_____

_____

_____

Step 4: Engage the Implementer in Guided Practice

- Have the implementer practice the intervention with your active support.
- Provide positive yet corrective feedback.
- Repeat guided practice until the implementer is ready to practice delivering the intervention independently.

"Now, it's your turn. How would you start the intervention? [*The implementer starts practicing the intervention.*] Exactly, so then next you will [*guide implementer on next steps*]. I really liked how you [*indicate something positive from his or her practice*]. Next time, consider [*explain how the implementer could do something differently*]. Let's see that in action again."

_____

_____

_____

_____

_____

(continued)

113

Step 5: Engage the Implementer in Independent Practice

- Have the implementer practice the intervention independently.
- Provide positive yet corrective feedback.
- Repeat independent practice until the implementer is prepared to deliver the intervention with fluency and fidelity.

> "Now, why don't you go through the intervention like you would if you were in the [*implementation setting*]. I really liked how you [*indicate something positive from their practice*]. Next time, consider [*explain how they could do something differently*]. Let's see that in action again."

_____

_____

_____

_____

_____

Step 6: Review the Meeting and Thank the Implementer

- Review the meeting discussion and decisions.
- Thank the implementer and close the meeting.

> "We discussed and practiced [*intervention*]. It seems like you're comfortable with the intervention and ready to go. Is that right? Any questions? [*Answer any questions.*] Thank you for meeting with me and, remember, you can always reach out with questions or for support."

_____

_____

_____

_____

_____

FOLLOW-UP CHECKLIST

✓	Have you . . .
☐	1. Reviewed the session notes to ensure that the strategy was delivered as planned?
☐	2. Updated the intervention plan and/or implementation plan, as needed?
☐	3. Checked in with the implementer following the meeting to touch base about implementation and answered his or her questions?

Fidelity Data Sheet for Direct Training

For each of the strategy steps, provide a rating of adherence (to what extent you covered each step) and of quality (how well you delivered each step) based on the following rubric.

Adherence	Quality
2 = All components of step delivered. 1 = Some components of step delivered. 0 = No components of step delivered.	2 = Step delivered in a smooth, natural manner, responsive to the implementer, and with appropriate nonverbal interaction. 1 = Step delivered with some aspects of quality. 0 = Step delivered without any aspects of quality.

Strategy Steps	Adherence	Quality
1. Explain the purpose of the session.		
2. Provide didactic intervention training.		
3. Demonstrate the intervention.		
4. Engage the implementer in guided practice.		
5. Engage the implementer in independent practice.		
6. Thank the implementer for the meeting.		

First, sum each column: _____   _____

12   12

Next, divide by number of steps to identify a percentage: = _____ %   = _____ %

CHAPTER 7

Participant Modeling and Role Play

WHAT ARE PARTICIPANT MODELING AND ROLE PLAY?

Participant modeling and role play are implementation supports in which the consultant demonstrates accurate intervention implementation and provides the implementer with an opportunity to practice intervention implementation with the consultant, observing and providing feedback (Box 7.1). The primary difference between the strategies is that par-

---

BOX 7.1. Participant Modeling and Role-Play Snapshot

 Who?	Implementers whose (1) fidelity data on intervention steps suggest that some or all of the steps are not implemented, and direct training has already been provided; or (2) session-level fidelity data indicate low levels of quality, even if adherence overall is adequate.
 What?	Demonstrating accurate intervention implementation and giving the implementer an opportunity to practice intervention implementation with the consultant, observing and providing feedback.
 Where? When?	*Participant modeling*: Will require two or three meetings, at least one of which is *in vivo*. *Role play*: Deliver it during a one-time session in a private meeting space.
 Why?	Each strategy provides the implementer with an opportunity to observe the consultant implementing intervention steps appropriately, and to practice with feedback until mastery is achieved. In participant modeling the practice occurs in the implementation context, and in role play the practice takes place in an analogue setting using mock scenarios.

---

ticipant modeling occurs partially *in vivo*, while implementation is occurring (e.g., during classroom instruction), whereas role play occurs entirely outside of the implementation context (e.g., in a classroom after school, in an office during the school day). Aside from this difference, the strategies are very similar. Both strategies are presented because some interventions and implementation challenges lend themselves to one strategy over the other.

Both participant modeling and role play begin with leading a review of the intervention and discussing the available intervention fidelity data and recipient outcome data. You will use the available intervention fidelity data to highlight intervention steps that are being implemented well, and to identify those that require additional practice. It is at this point that participant modeling and role play differ from one another in terms of where and how practice occurs. In participant modeling, you deliver the identified intervention steps to the recipient with the implementer watching. Then the implementer has an opportunity to practice those same steps with you observing and providing real-time feedback within the actual implementation context. In role play, first you play the role of implementer and deliver the identified intervention steps to the implementer, who plays the role of recipient. Then you and the implementer switch roles and the implementer practices delivering the same intervention steps to you, during which you provide real-time feedback outside of the implementation context. In both participant modeling and role play, you and the implementer will discuss the practice and may engage in additional practice, as necessary, until the implementer feels confident in his or her ability to implement the intervention independently.

RESEARCH ON PARTICIPANT MODELING AND ROLE PLAY

There is a vast body of research supporting the effectiveness of participant modeling as a behavior change strategy (Kazdin, 2013). Participant modeling has been used to help individuals acquire a wide range of behaviors resulting in changes such as improved parenting or caregiving behaviors (Minor, Minor, & Williams, 1983), reduced fears (Ollendick & King, 1998; Trijsburg, Jelicic, van den Broek, & Plekker, 1996), decreased stress (Romi & Teichman, 1998), improved diet (Winett, Kramer, Walker, Malone, & Lane, 1988), increased productivity (Newman & Tuckman, 1997), and decreased avoidance behaviors (Downs, Rosenthal, & Lichstein, 1988). Given its effectiveness as a behavior change strategy, it has also been applied to intervention implementation behaviors. Available evidence suggests that it can be effective in increasing teachers' implementation of behavioral interventions (Collier-Meek, Sanetti, et al., 2018; Sanetti & Collier-Meek, 2015; Sanetti et al., 2018).

Similarly, role play has a vast literature supporting its effectiveness as a behavior change strategy (Dobson, 2010). Role play has been used to help individuals improve their social (Chorpita, 2007; Frey, Elliott, & Miller, 2014; Yamamoto, Kagami, Ogura, & Isawa, 2013) and communication skills (Ammentorp, Kofoed, Laulaund, 2010) as well as decrease symptoms of anxiety (Braswell & Kendall, 2001; Chorpita, 2007) and depression (Chorpita, 2007). In addition to addressing social and emotional issues such as these, role play has been utilized as a way to support implementation of interventions. In professional development sessions role play is commonly used to provide performance-based learning experiences, which have been shown to increase the likelihood of skill acquisition (Joyce & Showers, 2002). Further, role play has been utilized in individual consulting or coaching contexts to improve educators' and parents' implementation of interventions (Collier-Meek, Sanetti, et al., 2018; Chorpita, 2007; Sterling-Turner et al., 2001).

HOW DO PARTICIPANT MODELING AND ROLE PLAY WORK?

Both participant modeling and role play are based on social learning theory (Bandura, 1977), which suggests that individuals can learn not only by engaging in a behavior and directly experiencing the consequence of that behavior (operant conditioning), but also by observing another person's behavior and the consequences, extracting information from those observations, and making decisions about their personal performance of the behavior (observational learning and imitation). Social learning theory is the basis of modeling, the process of observing an individual and imitating the behaviors (Kazdin, 2013). According to social learning theory, there are several elements necessary for someone to learn via modeling: (1) an actual person demonstrating the desired behavior, (2) a verbal description of the desired behavior, (3) attention to the modeled behavior, (4) an ability for the learner to retain the information about the modeled behavior, (5) an ability to reproduce the modeled behavior, and (6) motivation to imitate the behavior. It is important to note that learning can occur from modeling without the learner actually demonstrating the behavior; the learner's motivation to imitate the modeling is essential to the learner's actual demonstration of the learned behavior. **Although both strategies include modeling, participant modeling occurs during implementation, whereas role play occurs outside the implementation context.**

WHAT IMPLEMENTERS WILL BENEFIT
FROM PARTICIPANT MODELING OR ROLE PLAY?

Participant modeling and role play will benefit implementers when their (1) step-level fidelity data suggest that some or all of the intervention steps are not implemented and direct training has already been provided; or (2) session-level fidelity data indicate low levels of quality, even if adherence overall is adequate. These strategies can be especially critical when fidelity data indicate that preventive or less intrusive intervention steps are not being implemented, but responsive or more intrusive strategies are. In such instances, building the implementer's skill in the preventive or less intrusive intervention step may increase intervention effectiveness as well as the implementer–learner relationship. To decide between these two implementation support strategies, consider each strategy, the intervention being implemented, the implementer, and the context. For example, if intervention fidelity data suggest that an implementer is not implementing the consequence strategies for inappropriate behavior outlined in a student's behavior support plan, you would need to consider how often that behavior is emitted to determine if practicing *in vivo* is feasible. If it was a high-intensity but low-frequency behavior, then using role play may be more feasible and allow the implementer to gain confidence in his or her implementation ability prior to the next behavioral episode. Alternatively, if intervention fidelity data suggest that an implementer is struggling to implement an intervention to improve reading fluency during a small group, for example, it may be highly feasible to using participant modeling, assuming the implementer would welcome you into his or her classroom during instruction.

GETTING READY
FOR PARTICIPANT MODELING OR ROLE PLAY

Participant modeling and role play are both conversation- and modeling-based implementation support strategies that require some preparation ahead of time to allow for smooth and productive sessions with the implementer. Getting ready to deliver participant modeling or role play involves three steps, outlined in Box 7.2 and described below.

Step 1: Review the Intervention and Current Data

To prepare for participant modeling or role play, review the intervention and current data, if available. *Familiarize yourself with the intervention plan* so that you can fluently describe the how to and why of each intervention step as well as model and problem-solve delivering these steps with intervention fidelity. During the meeting, the implementer will refer to your expertise in the intervention and its implementation; be prepared to serve in this role. If not already completed as part of implementation planning or direct training, break the intervention into components (see Chapter 5). Also, *review the intervention goal and learner's progress* and *review intervention fidelity data* to be comfortable describing current patterns in these data sources (e.g., level, trend, variability, relationship between data

---

**BOX 7.2. Getting Ready to Deliver
Participant Modeling or Role Play**

1. Review the intervention and current data.
   - Familiarize yourself with the intervention plan.
   - Review the intervention goal and, using data, the learner's current progress.
   - Review intervention fidelity data.

2. Prepare for participant modeling and role play.
   - Read about participant modeling and role play.
   - Decide the order in which to model or role-play intervention steps.
   - Practice dialogue and modeling of intervention steps, as needed, to be comfortable at the meeting.

3. Identify session logistics.
   - Schedule participant modeling or role-play session(s).
   - Reach out to the implementer.
   - Bring participant modeling or role-play materials to the session.

sources). If possible, make graphs to illustrate this information, which can be used to identify intervention steps to model or role-play, and to focus discussion during the participant
modeling or role-play session (see Chapter 4). If the graphed intervention fidelity data indicate that none of the intervention steps has been implemented, then you will need to model
or role-play the entire intervention. However, if the data suggest only some of the intervention steps are implemented poorly or not at all, then you can focus your modeling and role
play on these specific intervention steps.

Step 2: Prepare for Participant Modeling and Role Play

To be comfortable delivering either strategy, carefully *read about participant modeling and
role play* and decide which strategy will allow you to best demonstrate the implementation of intervention steps that are currently not being implemented well or at all. Once you
have decided on a strategy, familiarize yourself with the strategy steps and talking points.
Confirm your understanding of the purpose of the strategy and each of the steps. With
the target intervention steps and implementation support strategy identified, *decide the
order in which to model or role-play intervention steps*. Intervention steps could be ordered
sequentially, by implementation scenario, or grouped by difficulty. For instance, if the intervention is brief or the steps build upon one another, it might make sense to simply practice
the intervention steps sequentially. If the implementer is struggling with implementation
during a particular time of day, then looking at a scenario relevant to that time of day or
modeling during that time of day may be most appropriate (see Quick Tip 7.1 below). If the
implementer is having difficulty with particularly challenging intervention steps, then focus
on steps grouped by difficulty. Prepare the list of intervention steps arranged in a tentative order for participant modeling or role play, to discuss with the implementer, as well
as any other necessary information or materials (e.g., graphs, reports, written intervention
plan, research). To *practice your dialogue and modeling of intervention steps*, review the
Participant Modeling Guide (Appendix 7.1) or Role-Play Guide (Appendix 7.2), intervention
fidelity data, intervention outcome data, and the intervention steps that will be modeled for
the implementer. This preparation will help you to maximize the strategy session and feel
comfortable addressing the implementer's concerns and needs.

Quick Tip 7.1. Drafting Scenarios

If you are implementing a role play, it is essential that the scenarios used during the role
plays are as authentic as possible. To use your meeting time with the implementer efficiently,
consider outlining possible scenarios to use during role plays prior to the meeting. Use the
available intervention fidelity data to inform which intervention steps need to be practiced.
Then consider what feedback you may have received from the implementer (e.g., what times of day are
challenging, what situations are challenging), as well as anything you have observed in the classroom
to inform the scenarios. Then present these to the implementer as examples of possible scenarios;
the implementer may (1) agree that the scenarios represent the times when he or she experiences
implementation challenges, (2) tweak the scenarios slightly, or (3) indicate that the scenarios are not
appropriate and suggest other options. Regardless, having scenario options available to which the
implementer may react can facilitate the efficient development of authentic examples for role play.

Step 3: Identify Session Logistics

Once ready, it is necessary to plan the session logistics. To *schedule a participant modeling or role-play session,* determine how long the meeting will last, when to hold the meeting, and how many sessions are needed to complete the strategy. Participant modeling will require three sessions; the first and third will occur outside of the implementation context and the second will occur *in vivo* during implementation. It is possible to have the three sessions in a single day (Session 1 before school, Session 2 during school, Session 3 after school), or it may be necessary to hold the sessions over a few days, based on scheduling. Hold the sessions as close together as possible to ensure that the implementer is ready for the implementation practice (Session 2) and able to describe the practice during the debriefing (Session 3). Role play typically occurs in one session outside the implementation setting. The duration of meetings for participant modeling and role play will be dependent on the type of intervention and the number of intervention steps to be practiced.

Decide who will be involved (e.g., primary implementer, potential collaborators). In some cases, there is more than one person implementing the intervention (e.g., paraprofessionals, school support professionals) or other stakeholders (e.g., case worker, parent), who may be interested in attending. Arrange where you will meet. For participant modeling, the first and third sessions need to be held in a quiet space that offers privacy for discussion; the second session will occur in the implementation setting. For role play, you will need a quiet space that offers privacy for discussion and the space and materials needed for realistic practice. Make sure time and location are feasible for implementer. *Reach out to the implementer* ahead of the participant modeling or role play session. If you think it would be helpful for the implementer to review any materials prior to the strategy meeting, provide those in advance (e.g., written list of intervention steps, sample intervention materials, research, data). *Bring participant modeling or role-play materials to the session.* For participant modeling or role play, these materials include the strategy guide (Appendix 7.1 or 7.2), written intervention plan, graphs of intervention fidelity and learner outcome data, and your list of intervention steps to be practiced.

PARTICIPANT MODELING AND ROLE PLAY STEP-BY-STEP

Participant modeling and role play involve modeling the intervention and providing an opportunity for the implementer to practice the intervention and receive feedback. The 11 steps of participant modeling and role play are provided in Box 7.3. Given that participant modeling and role play share six of the 11 steps, we describe the step-by-step delivery of both strategies together. Steps 1–4 and 9–11 are the same for both strategies; Steps 5–8 are different for each strategy and therefore are described separately.

The Participant Modeling Guide and the Role-Play Guide in Appendices 7.1 and 7.2, respectively, are separated in the two appendices for ease during implementation. Each guide includes the key objectives and sample language for each step, as well as space for recording implementer responses. This guide can be copied and used for delivering this implementation support in your practice. A description of each step of participant modeling and role play, including key objectives and quick tips for delivery, are provided in the following sections.

BOX 7.3. Participant Modeling and Role-Play Steps

Participant Modeling	Role Play
1. *Explain the purpose of the session.*	
2. *Discuss the intervention and the importance of implementation.*	
3. *Review the intervention steps in relation to intervention fidelity and learner outcome data.*	
4. *Identify the target intervention steps and set the goal.*	
5. Prepare for the *in vivo* exercise.	5. Discuss the practice scenarios.
6. Complete the *in vivo* demonstration.	6. Demonstrate the intervention step(s), with the implementer acting as the learner.
7. Facilitate *in vivo* supported practice.	7. Exchange feedback about the demonstration.
8. Facilitate *in vivo* independent practice.	8. The implementer role plays, with the consultant acting as the learner.
9. *Exchange feedback about the implementer's practice.*	
10. *Review the meeting and thank the implementer.*	

Step 1: Explain the Purpose of the Session

- Provide an overview of participant modeling or role play.
- Begin participant modeling or role play in an open, supportive manner.

To begin the first participant modeling or role-play session, explain the purpose of meeting to the implementer. Describe the purpose as a chance to review and practice implementation to ensure that he or she is comfortable delivering the intervention. Provide an overview of the participant modeling or role-play session by briefly reviewing the steps of the strategy (see Box 7.3). This way, the implementer will understand his or her role within these strategies and be prepared to practice implementation of the intervention with you.

Step 2: Discuss the Intervention and the Importance of Implementation

- Describe how the intervention addresses the current concern and will help the learner reach his or her goal.
- Explain how intervention implementation affects outcomes.

Describe the rationale for the intervention. That is, how does the intervention address the identified problem? Describe how the benefits of intervention implementation will likely help the learner reach his or her intervention goal. Discuss how high levels of intervention fidelity are related to more efficient improvements in learner outcome data. This should be a review for the implementer, as you (hopefully) discussed the rationale and importance of implementation during direct training. If so, this step should be brief. If you have not yet discussed these points with the implementer, then spend some time now reviewing the rationale and importance of implementation (see Chapter 6).

Step 3: Review the Intervention Steps in Relation to Intervention Fidelity and Learner Outcome Data

- Review intervention fidelity data.
- Provide positive feedback for consistently implemented steps and note intervention steps that appear to be more challenging to implement.
- Review learner data by highlighting progress toward the intervention goal.
- Link learner progress to intervention fidelity.

After describing the intervention rationale and the importance of implementation, review the intervention steps and make connections to the available intervention fidelity and learner outcome data. Provide praise for intervention steps that are consistently implemented. For intervention steps that are not implemented consistently or at all, review *how* each step is implemented, *why* each step is used, and *what* implementing each step will serve to accomplish. Ask the implementer questions throughout to elicit his or her perspective on intervention implementation (e.g., "Does that step rationale make sense?"; "What's challenging about that step?"). During this review, provide the implementer with the opportunity to make minor revisions to intervention steps, as needed. If revisions occur, update the intervention and implementation plan (see Chapter 5).

Step 4: Identify the Target Intervention Steps and Set the Goal

- Determine any intervention steps that are not being implemented consistently with the implementer.
- Set goals for practice.

With the implementer, decide which intervention steps will be targeted during the practice exercises. These intervention steps should be those that have not been implemented consistently with high quality. Use the review and discussion of intervention fidelity data in Step 3 as well as the list of intervention steps to practice that you developed before the session to guide the discussion, and also elicit suggestions from the implementer. It is most helpful to practice intervention steps that are an appropriate fit for modeling/role play and practice, rather than steps that are a single occurrence at the start of the implementation period (e.g., posting visual reminders in the classroom).

Once the target intervention steps are identified, collaborate with the implementer to identify general (e.g., a successful practice session) and specific (e.g., demonstrate strategies for a particularly difficult step) goals for the practice. You might say "What do you want to accomplish as you practice the intervention? Is there anything we should make sure to specifically address?" Use the previous discussion of the intervention fidelity data and other feedback to guide the development of goals.

Steps 5–8 differ for participant modeling and role play. Steps for participant modeling are described first, followed by those for role play.

Participant Modeling Step 5: Prepare for the In Vivo Exercise

- Determine the desired format for *in vivo* practice.
- Plan the logistics for entering/exiting the target setting.

Following selection of the target intervention steps, collaborate with the implementer to decide the format and logistics of the *in vivo* practice session, such as how you will enter and exit the target setting and the order of demonstrating the intervention steps. Suggest to the implementer that he or she may want to notify the learner and/or other people in the implementation context of your presence in advance.

Participant Modeling Step 6: Complete the In Vivo Demonstration

- Model how each of the targeted intervention steps should look and sound.
- Be mindful of body position, pace, and pronunciation.

The first step of the *in vivo* session is to model the delivery of the intervention steps according to plan. In doing so, make sure to attend to the adherence and quality of your implementation. In this way, the demonstration will make it clear to the implementer what high-quality implementation of the intervention looks like and how it can be feasibly and completely delivered with high quality. As you are in the implementation context, demonstrate how to respond to the learner and other individuals in keeping with the intervention plan. Be aware of body position, pace, and pronunciation to ensure that the implementer can see and hear you clearly.

Participant Modeling Step 7: Facilitate In Vivo Supported Practice

- Invite the implementer to practice the target intervention steps.
- Provide specific, positive, and corrective suggestions and feedback.
- Have the implementer practice with guidance until each step is mastered.
- Repeat modeling and guided practice as needed.

Following the demonstration of each target intervention step, invite the implementer to practice the steps with assistance. As the implementer practices, provide specific, positive, and corrective suggestions and feedback related to the adherence and quality of his or her implementation. Take care to provide this feedback in a positive and unobtrusive manner that is appropriate for the implementation context. To do so you might provide quiet encouragement ("Yes, nice explanation of the transition!"), small prompts ("OK, you just finished up that intervention step—what follow-up is needed?"), and gentle reminders ("Before you jump into that step, what should be done?"). Continue with the guided practice until the implementer has mastered each intervention step. If it is possible, based on the intervention and implementation context, repeat the practice and feedback process with targeted intervention steps, as needed. For example, intervention steps such as behavior-specific praise can be practiced repeatedly until mastery is achieved, whereas some intervention steps are implemented only once per class period and may not lend themselves to repeated practice.

Participant Modeling Step 8: Facilitate In Vivo Independent Practice

- The implementer practices the intervention steps without any feedback or support.

After supported practice, transition to an independent practice. That is, have the implementer deliver the intervention steps without your support. The transition between supported and independent practice may be clearly distinct ("I'll step back now so you can continue to deliver the intervention independently") or subtle, as you simply stop providing feedback. While the implementer independently delivers the intervention, take note of intervention steps implemented completely and with high quality, as well as those steps that might need further support.

Role-Play Step 5: Discuss the Practice Scenarios

- Ask the implementer to suggest some scenarios that he or she could use to practice the target intervention steps.
- If the implementer has difficulty identifying scenarios, suggest scenarios based on the intervention fidelity data.

Ask the implementer to suggest some scenarios in which to practice the target intervention steps. Having the implementer brainstorm scenarios provides an opportunity to practice implementation in realistic, and perhaps particularly challenging, situations. Also suggest scenarios that you identified before the session, based on the intervention fidelity data. The goal is to provide a demonstration of implementation that is the most useful to the implementer (i.e., meets his or her specific needs).

Role-Play Step 6: Demonstrate the Intervention Step(s), with the Implementer Acting as the Learner

- Demonstrate the intervention steps. During the demonstration, you may simply demonstrate delivering the intervention as planned, or you may describe what you are doing.

Demonstrate the target intervention steps. To do so, act as the "implementer" and have the implementer act as the "learner." You may demonstrate the intervention in one of two ways. One option is to describe the implementation behaviors as you enact them, while making mindful notes of both the adherence and quality of your implementation. For example, if you are demonstrating the step of moving closer to a student who is displaying problem behavior, say "Because I am seeing the student turning around and talking with a peer, I am moving toward him, while still paying attention to other students and providing behavior-specific praise to them for working quietly." These types of descriptions can help clarify intervention steps for the implementer. Another option is to simply demonstrate the intervention steps as planned without describing your behavior. Simple demonstration of the target intervention steps is particularly helpful when the implementer is struggling with delivering the intervention steps fluently, as this practice models the combination of intervention steps as it would occur during actual implementation. Either option may be used for different intervention steps, depending on such factors as the complexity of the intervention step and feedback from the implementer.

Role-Play Step 7: Exchange Feedback about the Demonstration

- Ask the implementer for feedback about the demonstration.
- Summarize and validate the implementer's perspective.
- Share your feedback about the demonstration, highlighting areas of relative ease and how you navigated the more difficult steps.
- Praise the implementer's role as the student.

Following the demonstration, engage the implementer in a dialogue about the demonstration. To do so, ask the implementer to share his or her feedback. For example, you may ask "What did you notice about how I responded to the problem behavior?" or "Did that intervention seem at all similar to how you were thinking about providing additional opportunities to respond?" Summarize the implementer's perspective on the demonstration and validate his or her feedback. Share your own thoughts about the demonstration by describing intervention steps that were easier or more challenging and strategies you used to implement the more difficult steps. Praise the implementer for acting as the learner during the demonstration.

Role-Play Step 8: The Implementer Role-Plays, with the Consultant Acting as the Learner

- Have the implementer role-play the intervention steps while you act as the learner.
- Observe his or her implementation closely, paying attention to verbal and nonverbal behavior as well as to moments of ease and difficulty.
- Encourage the implementer and provide prompts as necessary.

Have the implementer role-play an intervention step or group of steps while you act as the learner. In your role as learner, first act in a relatively straightforward manner, but then it may be helpful to demonstrate some typical challenging or distracting behaviors so that the implementer can have practice responding under conditions characteristic of his or her classroom. As the implementer practices the intervention steps, carefully observe his or her implementation. Make a note of intervention steps that appear relatively easy or difficult for the implementer to enact. Pay attention to both the adherence and quality of the implementer's delivery and consider both verbal and nonverbal behaviors. If necessary, encourage the implementer ("Yes, you've got it! Those were very clear directions") and provide prompts and reminders for accurate implementation ("OK, you just provided the directions—what's next?").

For participant modeling, Steps 9 and 10 may occur immediately after the *in vivo* practice, if the implementer's schedule allows (e.g., during a prep period immediately following the *in vivo* practice) or may occur in a third session.

Step 9: Exchange Feedback about the Implementer's Practice

- Ask the implementer to self-evaluate his or her practice.
- Provide constructive feedback, reinforce successes, and correct any implementation errors.

Debrief with the implementer following the *in vivo* practice or role play. Praise the implementer's efforts for delivering the intervention steps as planned. Ask the implementer which steps he or she delivered confidently and that went well. Provide praise for those steps. Also, ask the implementer which steps were more difficult to deliver. Summarize and validate the implementer's perspective about his or her implementation. Share your feedback about the *in vivo* practice or role play, staying positive and emphasizing intervention steps that were implemented successfully. Collaboratively with the implementer, brainstorm solutions to remaining areas of difficulty and prompt the implementer for his or her perspective. If needed, schedule more *in vivo* modeling sessions or repeat the role-play practice until the implementer has mastered all target intervention steps without your support.

Step 10: Review the Meeting and Thank the Implementer

- Review the implementation support provided.
- Thank the implementer and close the meeting.

To close a participant modeling or role-play session, review the implementation support goals and collaboratively determine whether they have been met. Ask the implementer if he or she has remaining questions about implementation or needs additional resources or support to maintain intervention implementation with fidelity. Provide positive feedback to the implementer and thank him or her for participating in participant modeling or role-play sessions.

FOLLOW-UP AFTER PARTICIPANT MODELING OR ROLE PLAY

To solidify the discussion and progress made during participant modeling or role play, we suggest that you engage in some activities after the session. Follow-up for either strategy involves three steps, outlined in Box 7.4 and described in the following material.

Review session notes to ensure that the strategy was delivered as planned. To do so, check the Participant Modeling Guide (Appendix 7.1) or the Role-Play Guide (Appendix

---

BOX 7.4. Follow-Up Steps after Participant Modeling or Role Play

1. Review session notes to ensure that the strategy was delivered as planned.
2. Update the intervention plan and/or implementation plan, as needed.
3. Check in with the implementer following the meeting to touch base about intervention fidelity and to answer any questions.

7.2) and complete a self-assessment using the Fidelity Data Sheet for Participant Modeling (Appendix 7.3) or the Fidelity Data Sheet for Role Play (Appendix 7.4) to see if you addressed each of the strategy steps. If you missed any steps, follow up with the implementer. It is important to make sure that the strategies were delivered as planned so that they have the most likelihood of impacting the implementer. If there were any adaptations made to the intervention plan because of participant modeling or role play, *update the intervention plan and/or implementation plan.* Share the updated materials with the implementer as soon as possible. Last, *check in with the implementer following the meeting to touch base about intervention fidelity and answer his or her questions.* This follow-up will ensure that the implementer feels comfortable delivering the intervention after the meeting and that his or her questions have been answered. Confirm that the implementer knows how to contact you with any questions about the intervention or its implementation.

SUMMARY

Participant modeling and role play are designed to increase implementer confidence and skill in implementation. To implement the strategy, the consultant and implementer discuss the rationale for implementing the selected intervention and identify target intervention steps for further practice. For participant modeling, the consultant demonstrates the target intervention steps in the target setting with the intervention recipient and facilitates guided and independent practice of the intervention steps. For role play, first the consultant and implementer identify common or challenging scenarios in the classroom. Next, the consultant demonstrates the target intervention steps, with the implementer acting as the recipient, followed by the recipient demonstrating the target intervention steps, with the consultant acting as the recipient. Both strategies conclude with the consultant and implementer debriefing about the implementation support strategy and determining if additional practice or support is needed. At the conclusion of the participant modeling or role-play session, the implementer should feel ready to deliver the intervention with high levels of intervention fidelity.

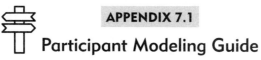

APPENDIX 7.1
Participant Modeling Guide

Consultant: _____ Implementer: _____

Learner: _____ Intervention: _____ Date: _____

Meeting 1 Date/Time: _____

Meeting 2 (*in vivo*) Date/Time: _____

Meeting 3 Date/Time: _____

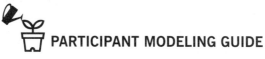 READINESS CHECKLIST

✓	Have you . . .
	1. Reviewed the intervention and current data?
☐	Familiarized yourself with the intervention plan?
☐	Reviewed intervention goal and, using data, the learner's current progress?
☐	Reviewed implementation data?
	2. Prepared for participant modeling?
☐	Read about participant modeling?
☐	Decided the order in which to model intervention steps?
☐	Practiced dialogue and modeling of intervention steps, as needed, to be comfortable at the meeting?
	3. Identified session logistics?
☐	Scheduled participant modeling?
☐	Reached out to the implementer?
☐	Brought participant modeling materials to the session?

PARTICIPANT MODELING GUIDE

Session 1

Step 1: Explain the Purpose of the Session

- Provide an overview of participant modeling or role play.
- Begin participant modeling or role play in an open, supportive manner.

(continued)

Following is an example of what you might say to explain the purpose of this session.

> "Today, we're here to discuss how implementing [*intervention*] has been going. Over two or three sessions we are going to talk about what's been working and what's been challenging. Then I'll model any intervention steps that have been challenging, and you'll practice implementing those steps with support from me. We will debrief about the practice and continue modeling and practicing until you believe you can implement [*intervention*] independently."

_____

_____

_____

Step 2: Discuss the Intervention and the Importance of Implementation

- Describe how the intervention addresses the current concern and will help the learner reach his or her goal.
- Explain how intervention implementation affects outcomes.

> "As you may recall from our initial training, we chose [*intervention*] because [*recipient*] needs support with [*target behavior/skill*] and [*intervention*] will address those concerns by [*rationale for intervention*]. Does that make sense? For any intervention to result in improved outcomes, the intervention has to be implemented as planned. I know that you want [*recipient*] to improve, and also that learning an intervention can be challenging, given all of your other responsibilities, so I am here to help!"

_____

_____

_____

Step 3: Review the Intervention Steps in Relation to Intervention Fidelity and Learner Outcome Data

- Review intervention fidelity data.
- Provide positive feedback for consistently implemented steps and note intervention steps that appear to be more challenging to implement.
- Review learner data by highlighting progress toward the intervention goal.
- Link learner progress to intervention fidelity.

> "How do you think [*recipient*] is responding to [*intervention*]? [*Summarize and validate response.*] First, let's take a look at how [*student*] has been doing. [*Show graphs.*] We had a goal for [*recipient*] of [*describe recipient goal*]. Based on the outcome data [*describe outcome data*], the [*recipient*] is on track/not on track to meet the goal. Now let's take a look at the implementation data we've collected. [*Show graphs and review implementation strengths.*] You've done an excellent job with [*describe implementation strengths*]. That's fantastic. [*Review implementation inconsistencies.*] I see that [*inconsistently implemented step(s)*] has been challenging to deliver on a regular basis. Is that right?"

_____

_____

_____

(continued)

Step 4: Identify the Target Intervention Steps and Set the Goal

- Determine any intervention steps that are not being implementing consistently with the implementer.
- Set goals for practice.

> "So, let's take a look at the challenging intervention steps. Do you agree that it would be beneficial to practice these steps more in [*target setting*]?"

_____

_____

_____

Step 5: Prepare for the In Vivo *Exercise*

- Determine the desired format for *in vivo* practice.
- Plan the logistics for entering/exiting the target setting.

> "Given that these are the steps we want to work on, let's talk about when it would be best to have an *in vivo* session and in what order we will practice the steps. Also, how would you like me to enter [*target setting*]? Do you think it's best for [*recipient*] to know that I'm coming?"

_____

_____

_____

Session 2: *In Vivo*

Step 6: Complete the In Vivo *Demonstration*

- Model how each of the targeted intervention steps should look and sound.
- Be mindful of body position, pace, and pronunciation.

> "Okay, now I will take over responsibility for implementing [*name intervention*]. I will try to describe why I am doing what I am doing as I go; if you have questions as you watch, write them down or ask me."

_____

_____

_____

(continued)

Step 7: Facilitate In Vivo *Supported Practice*

- Invite the implementer to practice the target intervention steps.
- Provide specific, positive, and corrective suggestions and feedback.
- Have the implementer practice with guidance until each step is mastered.
- Repeat modeling and guided practice as needed.

> "You've had a chance to see me implement the intervention steps, so why don't you go ahead and practice them now. I'm here to answer questions and support you."

_____

_____

_____

Step 8: Facilitate In Vivo *Independent Practice*

- The implementer practices the intervention steps without any feedback or support.

> "It looks like you really have got this! Nice job! Go ahead and implement the intervention on your own."

_____

_____

_____

Session 3

Step 9: Exchange Feedback about the Implementer's Practice

- Ask the implementer to self-evaluate his or her practice.
- Provide constructive feedback, reinforce successes, and correct any implementation errors.

> "You are really getting the hang of [*name intervention steps*], but I'd like to see you practice [*intervention steps*] a few more times. Focus on [*describe the change the implementer needs to make*]."

_____

_____

_____

(continued)

Step 10: Review the Meeting and Thank the Implementer

- Review the implementation support provided.
- Thank the implementer and close the meeting.

"We talked about parts of the intervention that have been going really well, and targeted some more challenging intervention steps for modeling and practice. You did a great job practicing those intervention steps, and you seem to be more fluent and confident in your implementation now. Does that seem accurate? Would you like to do more practice with my support? [*If yes, schedule another* in vivo *session.*] Improving your implementation is really going to help [*recipient*] reach his [*her*] intervention goal—great work! Do you have any questions? [*Answer any questions.*] Thank you for taking the time for these meetings and letting me into [*implementation context*]. Remember that you can always reach out with questions or for support."

_____

_____

_____

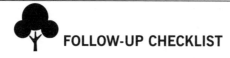 **FOLLOW-UP CHECKLIST**

✓	Have you . . .
☐	1. Reviewed session notes to ensure that the strategy was delivered as planned?
☐	2. Updated the intervention plan and/or implementation plan, as needed?
☐	3. Checked in with the implementer following the meeting to touch base about intervention fidelity and answer any questions?

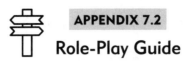

APPENDIX 7.2

Role-Play Guide

Consultant: _____   Implementer: _____

Learner: _____   Intervention: _____

Date/Time: _____

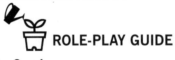

READINESS CHECKLIST

✓	Have you . . .
1. Reviewed the intervention and current data?	
☐	Familiarized yourself with the intervention plan?
☐	Reviewed intervention goal and, using data, the learner's current progress?
☐	Reviewed intervention fidelity data?
2. Prepared for participant modeling?	
☐	Read about role play?
☐	Decided the order in which to role-play intervention steps?
☐	Practiced dialogue and modeling of intervention steps, as needed, to be comfortable at the meeting?
3. Identified session logistics?	
☐	Scheduled role-play session(s)?
☐	Reached out to the implementer?
☐	Brought role-play materials to the session?

ROLE-PLAY GUIDE

Step 1: Explain the Purpose of the Session

- Provide an overview of participant modeling or role play.
- Begin participant modeling or role play in an open, supportive manner.

"Today, we're here to discuss how implementing [intervention] has been going. During our meeting today, we will talk about what's been working and also about those scenarios that are particularly challenging. Then we'll role-play those scenarios, first with me as the implementer and you as the student, and then with you as the implementer and me as the student. We'll end by debriefing

(continued)

about the practice and continue role-playing and practicing until you believe you can implement [*intervention*] independently. Any questions?"

_____

_____

_____

Step 2: Discuss the Intervention and the Importance of Implementation

- Describe how the intervention addresses the current concern and will help the learner reach his or her goal.
- Explain how intervention implementation affects outcomes.

"As you may recall from our initial training, we chose [*intervention*] because [*recipient*] needs support with [*target behavior/skill*], and [*intervention*] will address those concerns by [*rationale for intervention*]. Does that make sense? For any intervention to result in improved outcomes, the intervention has to be implemented as planned. I know you want [*recipient*] to improve, and also that learning an intervention can be challenging, given all of your other responsibilities, so I am here to help!"

_____

_____

_____

Step 3: Review the Intervention Steps in Relation to Intervention Fidelity and Learner Outcome Data

- Review intervention fidelity data.
- Provide positive feedback for consistently implemented steps and note intervention steps that appear to be more challenging to implement.
- Review learner data by highlighting progress toward the intervention goal.
- Link learner progress to intervention fidelity.

"How do you think [*recipient*] is responding to [*intervention*]? [*Summarize and validate response.*] First, let's take a look at how [*recipient*] has been doing. [*Show graphs.*] We had a goal for [*recipient*] of [*describe recipient goal*]. Based on the outcome data [*describe outcome data*], the [*recipient*] is on track/not on track to meet the goal. Now let's take a look at the implementation data we've collected. [*Show graphs and review implementation strengths.*] You've done an excellent job with [*describe implementation strengths*]. That's fantastic. [*Review implementation inconsistencies.*] I see that [*inconsistently implemented step(s)*] has been challenging to deliver on a regular basis. Is that right?"

_____

_____

_____

(continued)

Step 4: Identify Target Intervention Steps and Set the Goal

- Determine any intervention steps that are not being implemented consistently with the implementer.
- Set goals for practice.

  "So, let's take a look at the challenging intervention steps. Do you agree that it would be beneficial to role-play these steps?"

_____

_____

_____

Step 5: Discuss the Practice Scenarios

- Ask the implementer to suggest some scenarios that he or she could use to practice the target intervention steps.
- If the implementer has difficulty identifying scenarios, suggest scenarios based on the intervention fidelity data.

  "We need to come up with some scenarios to provide a context for our role plays. Think about implementing this intervention. What situations are the most challenging? [*Summarize and validate responses.*] OK, why don't we use this/those scenario/s for the first role play." [*Describe the scenario*].

_____

_____

_____

Step 6: Demonstrate the Intervention Step(s), with the Implementer Acting as the Learner

- Demonstrate the intervention steps. During the demonstration, you may simply demonstrate delivering the intervention as planned, or you may describe what you are doing.

  "I would say to the student, 'I am providing verbal praise because you raised your hand without calling out' [*adherence*]. I said 'Nice job raising your hand and waiting to be called on,' not 'Good job,' so that the praise was specific and immediate, which is more effective' [*quality*]."

_____

_____

_____

(continued)

Step 7: Exchange Feedback about the Demonstration

- Ask the implementer for feedback about the demonstration.
- Summarize and validate the implementer's perspective.
- Share your feedback about the demonstration, highlighting areas of relative ease and how you navigated the more difficult steps.
- Praise the implementer's role as the student.

> "How you think that went? [*Summarize and validate responses.*] I thought that [*intervention steps*] came more easily [*provide rationale, e.g., they are cued*]. I used [*describe how you managed more challenging steps*] to help me with [*intervention steps*]. You did a great job as the student!"

_____

_____

_____

Step 8: The Implementer Role-Plays, with the Consultant Acting as the Learner

- Have the implementer role-play the intervention steps while you act as the learner.
- Observe his or her implementation closely, paying attention to verbal and nonverbal behavior as well as to moments of ease and difficulty.
- Encourage the implementer and provide prompts as necessary.

> "All right, it is your turn to practice implementing, and I'll pretend to be the student. We came up with several scenarios; which one would you like to use first?"

_____

_____

_____

Step 9: Exchange Feedback about the Implementer's Practice

- Ask the implementer to self-evaluate his or her practice.
- Provide constructive feedback, reinforce successes, and correct any implementation errors.

> "So, how do you think that went? What do you think went well? Which steps were more challenging? [*Summarize and validate responses.*] I saw that you did [*describe intervention steps*] really well. Excellent work. It seemed as though [*describe intervention steps*] were still a little challenging. For example, [*provide specific corrective feedback*]. What can we do to make [*intervention steps*] less challenging?" [*Consider role-playing additional scenarios.*]

_____

_____

_____

(continued)

Step 10: Review the Meeting and Thank the Implementer

- Review the implementation support provided.
- Thank the implementer and close the meeting.

"We talked about parts of the intervention that have been going really well, and targeted some more challenging intervention steps for role playing. You did a great job practicing those intervention steps, and you seem to be more fluent and confident in your implementation now. Does that seem accurate? Would you like to role-play more? [*If yes, schedule another meeting.*] Improving your implementation is really going to help [*recipient*] reach her [*his*] intervention goal—great work! Do you have any questions? [*Answer any questions.*] Thank you for taking the time to meet with me to practice implementation. Remember that you can always reach out for questions or support."

_____

_____

_____

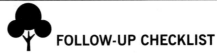 **FOLLOW-UP CHECKLIST**

✓	Have you . . .
☐	1. Reviewed session notes to ensure that the strategy was delivered as planned?
☐	2. Updated the intervention plan and/or implementation plan, as needed?
☐	3. Checked in with the implementer following the meeting to touch base about intervention fidelity and answer any questions?

Fidelity Data Sheet for Participant Modeling

For each of the strategy steps, provide a rating of adherence (to what extent you covered each step) and of quality (how well you delivered each step) based on the following rubric.

Adherence	Quality
2 = All components of step delivered. 1 = Some components of step delivered. 0 = No components of step delivered.	2 = Step delivered in a smooth, natural manner, responsive to the implementer, and with appropriate nonverbal interaction. 1 = Step delivered with some aspects of quality. 0 = Step delivered without any aspects of quality.

Strategy Steps	Adherence	Quality
1. Explain the purpose of the session.		
2. Discuss the intervention and the importance of implementation.		
3. Review the intervention steps in relation to intervention fidelity and learner outcome data.		
4. Identify the target intervention steps and set the goal.		
5. Prepare for the *in vivo* exercise.		
6. Complete the *in vivo* demonstration.		
7. Facilitate *in vivo* supported practice.		
8. Facilitate *in vivo* independent practice.		
9. Exchange feedback about the implementer's practice.		
10. Review the meeting and thank the implementer.		

First, sum each column: _____   _____

20   20

Next, divide by number of steps to identify a percentage: = _____ %   = _____ %

Fidelity Data Sheet for Role Play

For each of the strategy steps, provide a rating of adherence (to what extent you covered each step) and of quality (how well you delivered each step) based on the following rubric.

Adherence	Quality
2 = All components of step delivered. 1 = Some components of step delivered. 0 = No components of step delivered.	2 = Step delivered in a smooth, natural manner, responsive to the implementer, and with appropriate nonverbal interaction. 1 = Step delivered with some aspects of quality. 0 = Step delivered without any aspects of quality.

Strategy Steps	Adherence	Quality
1. Explain the purpose of the session.		
2. Discuss the intervention and the importance of implementation.		
3. Review the intervention steps in relation to intervention fidelity and learner outcome data.		
4. Identify the target intervention steps and set the goal.		
5. Discuss the practice scenarios.		
6. Demonstrate the intervention step(s), with the implementer acting as the learner.		
7. Exchange feedback about the demonstration.		
8. The implementer role-plays, with the consultant acting as the learner.		
9. Exchange feedback about the implementer's practice.		
10. Review the meeting and thank the implementer.		

First, sum each column: _____ _____

20 20

Next, divide by number of steps to identify a percentage: = _____% = _____%

CHAPTER 8

Self-Monitoring

WHAT IS SELF-MONITORING?

Self-monitoring is a bit different than the other implementation supports described in this book. Instead of the focus being on the activities that occur during the session between you and the implementer, the thrust of this strategy is a new activity in which the implementer will engage *after* meeting with you. That is, through meeting with you, the implementer will learn why and how to self-monitor his or her intervention fidelity (see Box 8.1). It turns

BOX 8.1. Self-Monitoring Snapshot

 Who? Implementers who are beginning implementation or struggling with performance-based deficits, are concerned about remembering to deliver the intervention, and willing to engage in in self-monitoring.

 What? The development of a tool and plan for the implementer to monitor his or her own intervention implementation.

 Where? When? Prepare during a one-time session in a private meeting space, then calibrate the implementer's self-monitoring by observing and comparing ratings, and have the implementer self-monitor after subsequent intervention implementation.

 Why? It helps the implementer pay more attention to his or her implementation behavior, which tends to lead to improvements in intervention fidelity.

out that simply monitoring intervention fidelity can lead to an increase in intervention fidelity. This same logic is why self-monitoring is often an intervention for students; it prompts and reinforces them for engaging in desired behavior (e.g., academic engagement; Briesch & Chafouleas, 2009; Fantuzzo & Polite, 1990). In the adult realm, many monitor desired behaviors, such as food intake or trips to the gym (Baker & Kirschenbaum, 1993; Kitsantas, 2000). When you monitor a desired behavior, you pay more attention to that behavior and, by doing so, tend to improve your behavior.

Self-monitoring alone, however, will not be sufficient for some implementers to change their behavior. Self-monitoring can involve several adaptations that might make this form of implementation support more relevant for these implementers (Cooper et al., 2007). For instance, there are several proactive, or antecedent-based, modifications that can be combined with self-monitoring to remind the implementer about the intervention steps. Other adaptations follow self-monitoring and include self-evaluation (i.e., compare self-monitoring and/or intervention fidelity data to a predetermined intervention fidelity goal), reinforcement (i.e., provide a pleasant consequence after meeting a self-monitoring and/or intervention fidelity goal), and performance feedback (i.e., meeting to review self-monitoring, intervention fidelity, and student outcome data; see Chapter 10). These modifications are described in an upcoming section, "Adaptations to Self-Monitoring," and the rest of the chapter describes the general self-monitoring process.

RESEARCH ON SELF-MONITORING

Self-monitoring has been well researched as a behavior change strategy for learners (e.g., Briesch & Chafouleas, 2009; Fantuzzo & Polite, 1990). Its effectiveness and low-intensity nature combined with the impetus provided by the intervention activity on the individual makes it well suited to facilitate implementer behavior change as well. Several studies have demonstrated that self-monitoring can effectively increase accurate administration of curriculum-based measurement and associated instructional decisions (Allinder, Bolling, Oats, & Gagnon, 2000), rates of behavior-specific praise (Simonsen et al., 2013; Thompson, Marchant, Anderson, Prater, & Gibb, 2012), and the implementation of discrete trial training (Belfiore, Fritts, & Herman, 2008), learning trials (Lylo & Lee, 2013), behavior support plans (Mouzakitis et al., 2015), and token economies (Petscher & Bailey, 2006; Plavnick et al., 2010). In some of these investigations, self-monitoring was most effective when combined with other components, such as performance feedback (Mouzakitis et al., 2015) or coaching (Thompson et al., 2012). These studies suggest that implementers can feasibly self-monitor and that doing so regularly can increase their intervention fidelity.

HOW DOES SELF-MONITORING WORK?

As we've discussed throughout this book, behavior change (e.g., learning a new intervention and delivering it with fidelity) can be challenging. We can alter the environment to increase the likelihood of behavior change by, for instance, planfully contextualizing the intervention through implementation planning (Chapter 5) or providing praise and suggestions about intervention fidelity data through performance feedback (Chapter 10). Self-monitoring works by giving implementers the opportunity to alter their own environments (Cooper et al., 2007). This happens in one of two possible ways: by altering variables to make the probability of the desired behavior more likely (i.e., controlling response) or by altering variables to provide a consequence after the behavior occurs to change the likelihood of behavior in the future (i.e., controlled response; Cooper et al., 2007). Stated more directly, self-monitoring is thought to impact individuals' behavior by (1) prompting them to, or reminding them of, the desired behavior (making it more likely that they will engage in the behavior) and (2) providing a positive consequence of the desired behavior (e.g., feeling proud of engaging in the desired behavior, decreasing guilt about desired behavior, receiving a planned reward for engaging in the desired behavior). Although the way that self-monitoring works is unknown, as it is difficult to evaluate exactly how these internal processes operate, self-monitoring has been found to be an effective intervention for implementation and other desired behaviors (Baker & Kirschenbaum, 1993; Briesch & Chafouleas, 2009; Fantuzzo & Polite, 1990; Simonsen et al., 2013).

WHAT IMPLEMENTERS WILL BENEFIT FROM SELF-MONITORING?

Self-monitoring is an adaptable form of implementation support that can be helpful for many implementers. Self-monitoring can be started at the onset of intervention implementation or added during the course of the implementation process, if intervention fidelity is low. Although we suggest that all implementers receive implementation planning and direct training at the onset of intervention implementation, in some cases, self-monitoring can be helpful to add to this support process. The addition of self-monitoring may be warranted if the implementer indicates that he or she is concerned about remembering to deliver the intervention, if the intervention occurs infrequently (so that the implementer may need prompting to deliver the intervention steps), or if the implementer expresses interest in monitoring his or her intervention fidelity. When provided during the course of intervention implementation, self-monitoring is best suited to target performance-based deficits (i.e., the implementer has the skills to implement the intervention, but is not consistently demonstrating them). When deciding among performance-building implementation supports, consider self-monitoring if the implementer seems to struggle to remember when and how to deliver the intervention with fidelity, but seems generally onboard with intervention implementation. Also, consider whether the implementer would be willing and open to take on this new responsibility.

GETTING READY FOR SELF-MONITORING

Like other strategies, self-monitoring includes meeting with the implementer, but more so, it involves key preparation and follow-up activities. Getting ready to deliver self-monitoring involves three steps, outlined in Box 8.2 and described in the following material.

BOX 8.2. Getting Ready for Self-Monitoring

1. Review the intervention and current data.
   - Familiarize yourself with the intervention plan.
   - Review the intervention fidelity data sheet that you are using to monitor implementation (see Chapter 3).
   - Review the intervention goal and, using data, the learner's current progress.
   - Evaluate the intervention fidelity data.

2. Prepare for self-monitoring.
   - Read about self-monitoring.
   - Create the first draft of the self-monitoring tool.
   - Practice dialogue, as needed, to be comfortable at the meeting.

3. Identify session logistics.
   - Schedule the self-monitoring session.
   - Reach out to the implementer.
   - Bring self-monitoring materials to the session.

Step 1: Review the Intervention and Current Data

To prepare for self-monitoring, review the intervention and current data, if available. *Familiarize yourself with the intervention plan* so that you are able to clearly discuss it step-by-step and create the self-monitoring tool. *Review the intervention fidelity data sheet that you are using to monitor implementation (see Chapter 3)*, as it will provide an initial sample template for your self-monitoring tool. If you are preparing for self-monitoring to occur during intervention implementation, *review the intervention goal and the learner's progress and evaluate the intervention fidelity data* so that you can ascertain and describe current patterns in these data sources (e.g., level, trend, variability, relationship between data sources) to the implementer during the meeting. You might also use these data to inform the development of the self-monitoring tool. For instance, if the implementer is struggling to deliver specific intervention steps, you might include directions or reminders about how to deliver those steps on the form or focus the form solely on these challenging intervention steps.

Step 2: Prepare for Self-Monitoring

To be comfortable delivering this strategy, carefully *read about self-monitoring* and familiarize yourself with the strategy steps and talking points. Consider the potential adaptations to self-monitoring and decide if and what adaptations you might want to incorporate. Confirm your understanding of the purpose of the strategy and each of the steps. In particular, make sure to note the preparation and follow-up activities specific to this form of implementation support. To make the session with the implementer as efficient as possible, *create the first draft of the self-monitoring tool.* To do so, refer to the steps for documenting intervention fidelity in Chapter 3: (1) List the intervention steps, (2) choose the assessment method, (3) identify a rating option, and (4) prepare to summarize data. A self-report intervention fidelity tool is basically a self-monitoring form. See Quick Tip 8.1: Creating a Self-Monitoring Tool on page 146 for guidance about this process, look at examples in Chapter 11, and check the Preparation Worksheet for Self-Monitoring in Appendix 8.3 to make sure it is ready. During the session with the implementer, you may make modifications to the self-monitoring tool. So, in addition to the drafted self-monitoring tool, it can be helpful to bring a few options (e.g., different rating scales) to illustrate how the tool might be organized differently. Last, to *practice your dialogue*, review the Self-Monitoring Guide (see Appendix 8.1), and, if applicable, review intervention fidelity and learner outcome data. This preparation will help you to maximize the strategy session.

Step 3: Identify Session Logistics

Once ready, it is necessary to plan the session logistics. To *schedule self-monitoring*, determine how long the meeting will last, when to hold the meeting, and how many sessions are needed to complete the strategy. Plan to meet for approximately 20–30 minutes. Decide who will be involved (e.g., primary implementer, potential collaborators). In some cases, there is more than one person implementing the intervention (e.g., paraprofessionals, school support professionals) or other stakeholders (e.g., case worker, parent) who may be interested in attending. Arrange where you will meet. You will need a quiet space that offers privacy for discussion. Make sure time and location are feasible for the implementer. *Reach out to the implementer* ahead of the self-monitoring session. If you think it would be helpful for the implementer to review any materials prior to the strategy meeting, provide those in advance (e.g., written list of intervention steps, sample intervention materials, research, data). *Bring self-monitoring materials* to the session, including the Self-Monitoring Guide (see Appendix 8.1), the Preparation Worksheet for Self-Monitoring (see Appendix 8.3), written intervention plan, the intervention fidelity form (see Chapter 3 for how to develop), self-monitoring tool draft(s), and, if applicable, graphs of intervention fidelity and learner outcome data.

SELF-MONITORING STEP-BY-STEP

As noted previously, self-monitoring is primarily effective because of what the implementer does *after* this meeting—that is, ideally, rates his or her own intervention fidelity on an ongoing basis. However, this session can ensure only that the implementer is *prepared* to monitor his or her intervention fidelity. The seven steps of a self-monitoring session are listed in Box 8.3. The Self-Monitoring Guide at the end of this chapter (Appendix 8.1) includes the steps, key objectives, and sample language, as well as space for recording the implementer's responses. This guide can be copied and used for delivering this implementation support in your practice. Use this guide, in addition to the Preparation Worksheet for Self-Monitoring (Appendix 8.3), also included at the end of this chapter. A description of the steps for the self-monitoring session, including key objectives and quick tips for delivery, are provided in the following sections.

BOX 8.3. Self-Monitoring Steps

1. Explain the purpose of the session.
2. Review the intervention and available intervention fidelity data.
3. Review and finalize the self-monitoring tool.
4. Practice self-monitoring.
5. Decide whether to incorporate any self-monitoring adaptations.
6. Make a plan for collecting self-monitoring data.
7. Review the meeting and thank the implementer.

Quick Tip 8.1. Creating a Self-Monitoring Form

Self-monitoring forms can look very different and can be customized to best fit the intervention, the current intervention fidelity data, and the implementer. As you go about developing a self-monitoring form, here are some suggestions:

- Consider starting with the intervention fidelity tool that you've already developed. The benefits of this approach are that you will be able to directly compare data collected via the self-monitoring form to the intervention fidelity tool. Make any necessary modifications to ensure that the wording is user-friendly and that the measure is feasible to complete (e.g., change intervals from 15 seconds to 1 minute).
- Use the intervention fidelity data and your knowledge about the intervention (and its research base!) to target your self-monitoring form. In some cases, it is not necessary for the form to include all intervention steps. In fact, you may decide just to have the implementer monitor particular steps that are challenging but important for learner outcomes. Once these intervention steps are delivered regularly, you may decide to add different intervention steps on the form.
- Write the self-monitoring form from the perspective of the implementer. That is, use wording such as "I provided . . ." and "I engaged in. . . ."
- Make sure that the self-monitoring form is feasible for the implementer to complete in the midst of his or her other responsibilities. For instance, make sure that the number of items and time intervals are reasonable.
- Some implementers might want to publically post the self-monitoring form to remind themselves to self-monitor and to make the form easy to complete. Make the self-monitoring form visually appealing! Include pictures and positive prompts!
- It can be tempting to rate intervention steps as fully completed when actually they have not been done as planned. To proactively address this issue, consider providing a range of rating options (e.g., completed as planned, completed but not as planned, not completed) that allow the implementer to comfortably admit when an intervention step was skipped or delivered in some modified manner.
- In addition to adherence, consider including space for quality and exposure ratings. This will allow the implementer to monitor whether he or she delivers intervention steps as planned, how well these steps are delivered, and for how long.
- Include a space for narrative comments. This space will encourage implementers to write a brief note as a reminder about why intervention steps were or were not delivered as planned and what, if any, modifications were made.
- Make sure the form is accompanied by a how-to guide that explains the intervention steps; how to deliver them with full adherence, quality, and exposure; and the rating options. This information will help the implementer rate him- or herself accurately.

Step 1: Explain the Purpose of the Session

- Provide an overview of self-monitoring.
- If available, highlight learner outcome data.
- Begin the session in an open, supportive manner.

As the self-monitoring session begins, provide an overview to help the implementer understand this strategy and what his or her role will be. Explain that self-monitoring is a low-intensity strategy that helps individuals pay attention to important new behaviors (e.g., eating healthily, going to the gym, implementing an intervention). If learner outcome data are available, highlight the need to ensure that the intervention is delivered as planned to help the learner stay on track to meet his or her goal. Explain that you will be reviewing the intervention and developing a self-monitoring plan together. Consider asking the implementer if he or she has any initial questions or concerns or would like to add any more items to the agenda. This approach can help set a tone of collaboration and active engagement during the session.

Step 2: Review Intervention and Available Intervention Fidelity Data

- Describe the how and why of each intervention step.
- If available, highlight intervention fidelity data.

Carefully describe each intervention step and the available intervention fidelity data. At the end of this discussion, the implementer should understand the purpose of each intervention step and how to implement it correctly. To do so, review each intervention step, providing detailed instructions about how to carry out the step and making sure to address the adherence, quality, and exposure, as applicable. Emphasize *why* each intervention step is important and *what* it is designed to accomplish by describing relevant theory and research. Make the link between the intervention steps and the effectiveness of the intervention for the learner. If available, use intervention fidelity data to highlight the intervention steps. Provide praise for steps consistently delivered (e.g., "You've done a really nice job with this step . . .") and convey understanding and provide greater detail about steps that were delivered inconsistently (e.g., "It seems like this step has been challenging . . .").

Step 3: Review and Finalize the Self-Monitoring Tool

- Review the draft of the self-monitoring tool and the potential rating options.
- Collaborate to finalize the self-monitoring tool.

Next, turn from describing the why and how of intervention steps to how the implementer will self-monitor his or her intervention implementation. Use the draft of the self-monitoring tool that you developed for the meeting to facilitate this discussion. Explain how to complete each self-monitoring item and why you thought the implementer could rate the intervention steps in this manner. Describe other potential rating options. Elicit the implementer's opinion about the clarity of the items and the rating options. Through discussion, refine the items to make sure each sufficiently addresses the implementation of each intervention step and is understandable and easy for the implementer to complete regularly. At the end of this step, you should have a collaboratively refined self-monitoring tool. Use the Preparation Worksheet for Self-Monitoring (Appendix 8.3) to make sure the form that addresses all the intervention steps (or at least those in need of improvement as indicated by intervention fidelity data); includes ratings for adherence, quality, and/or exposure; and is easy to understand, feasible to complete, and visually appealing. You may not be able to make all updates during the meeting, but make sure to take comprehensive notes to provide the final self-monitoring tool to the implementer shortly after the meeting.

Step 4: Practice Self-Monitoring

- Model how to self-monitor intervention steps.
- Have the implementer practice completing the form.
- Provide positive yet corrective feedback.

Model how you would rate each intervention step on the self-monitoring form. To demonstrate, (1) provide examples of how you might rate particular steps (e.g., "I would rate this step as fully completed if I . . ."), or (2) explain how you might self-monitor following a particular scenario (e.g., "If during our morning reading block, I had been able to provide several prompts but few praise statements . . ."). Next, engage the implementer in practice. To do so, offer a scenario and then ask how he or she would rate the intervention steps. Provide feedback to the implementer about the self-ratings. Reinforce accuracy and correct any misunderstandings about intervention steps or ratings. Some implementers will benefit from practice and feedback. Repeat the practice and feedback process until the implementer is able to accurately complete the self-monitoring form.

Step 5: Decide Whether to Incorporate Any Self-Monitoring Adaptations

- Explain adaptations to the self-monitoring tool and the potential benefits.
- Decide if and which adaptations will be included.

Self-monitoring can be effective in its own right (e.g., Simonsen et al., 2013) or when combined with other adaptations (e.g., Mouzakitis et al., 2015). We suggest that you consider incorporating at least some adaptations because they require minimal effort and have the potential to increase the likelihood that self-monitoring will be completed regularly. Review Table 8.1 for the list of potential adaptations (see page 151) and see the "Adaptations to Self-Monitoring" section beginning on page 150 for more information (e.g., how to implement, when to incorporate). Use the Preparation Worksheet for Self-Monitoring (Appendix 8.3) to document which, if any, potential adaptations you decide to incorporate and include any relevant details (e.g., potential goal, data for reinforcement).

Step 6: Make a Plan for Collecting Self-Monitoring Data

- Decide when and how often the implementer will self-monitor.
- Make a plan to calibrate self-monitoring ratings.

The crux of this implementation support applies to what occurs after this session, so it is important to outline the plan together. First, decide when and how often the implementer will self-monitor. In most cases, the implementer should plan to self-monitor after each time he or she delivers the intervention (e.g., daily, three or four times per week). This frequency is recommended because self-monitoring serves as a prompt to deliver the intervention with fidelity, and it is relatively feasible to do (e.g., brief to complete). If the implementer self-monitors consistently, and intervention fidelity improves, it may be appropriate to reduce the schedule of self-monitoring. Depending on the incorporated adaptations, it may be helpful to outline the schedule for evaluation, reinforcement, or performance feedback. Record the decisions on the Preparation Worksheet for Self-Monitoring (Appendix 8.3).

Next, explain to the implementer that you would like to calibrate his or her self-monitoring ratings *in vivo*. To do so, you will observe his or her implementation, and both you and the implementer will complete the self-monitoring tool. Then you will compare the self-monitoring ratings and discuss areas of agreement and disagreement to ensure that you are both on the same page about what constitutes intervention fidelity. Be positive yet corrective in your feedback. Answer any questions from the implementer. Focus on facilitating a feeling of confidence in the implementer with intervention implementation and a feeling of comfort in completing the self-monitoring tool. Determine one or more dates for this self-monitoring calibration and record this on the Preparation Worksheet for Self-Monitoring (Appendix 8.3).

Step 7: Review the Meeting and Thank the Implementer

- Review the discussion and decisions made in the meeting.
- Thank the implementer and close the meeting.

The implementer should leave this session with a solid understanding of the intervention and the plan for self-monitoring. Review the meeting and provide positive feedback to the implementer about his or her willingness to self-monitor. Highlight the link between the intervention steps, intervention fidelity, and positive changes in outcomes for the learner. Before closing the session, ask the implementer if he or she has any remaining questions about the intervention or about self-monitoring. End the meeting by thanking the implementer for engaging with you during the self-monitoring practice and mention that you will see the implementer soon when you calibrate his or her self-monitoring ratings.

FOLLOW-UP AFTER SELF-MONITORING

The key part of self-monitoring is what you do after the session: namely, rate your own intervention fidelity as planned. However, you have some follow-up activities as well, some of which were outlined during the meeting. Follow-up after self-monitoring involves four steps, outlined in Box 8.4 and described below.

> ## BOX 8.4. Self-Monitoring Follow-Up Steps
>
>
>
> 1. Review session notes and completed the Fidelity Data Sheet for Self-Monitoring (Appendix 8.2) to ensure that the strategy was delivered as planned.
> 2. Provide the agreed-upon version of the self-monitoring form and the Preparation Worksheet for Self-Monitoring (Appendix 8.3).
> 3. Calibrate the implementer's self-monitoring.
> 4. Check in with the implementer following the meeting to touch base about intervention fidelity and self-monitoring and to answer any questions.

Review your session notes to ensure that the strategy was delivered as planned. To do so, check the Self-Monitoring Guide (Appendix 8.1) and complete a self-assessment using the Fidelity Data Sheet for Self-Monitoring (Appendix 8.2) to see if you addressed each of the strategy steps. If you missed any steps, follow up with the implementer. It is important to make sure that the strategies were delivered as planned so that they have the most likelihood of impacting the implementer. *Provide the agreed-upon version of the self-monitoring form and the Preparation Worksheet for Self-Monitoring* (Appendix 8.3) to the implementer. This will ensure that he or she has the necessary materials to engage in self-monitoring as well as the specifics about the plan. *Calibrate the implementer's self-monitoring* by comparing it to intervention fidelity data. To do so, you will need to collect intervention fidelity data and then compare it to the implementer's ratings on the self-monitoring form. It is not necessary for ratings to match exactly, but they should be very close (i.e., approximately same level of intervention fidelity, same strengths and weaknesses). A match between these data sources will give you confidence that the implementer is accurately critiquing his or her own intervention fidelity. It may be necessary to compare intervention fidelity data to self-monitoring data several times before the implementer is able to accurately rate his or her own implementation. If you compare these data sources and find that the ratings are contradictory, provide positive yet corrective feedback to the implementer to support him or her to more accurately rate his or her intervention fidelity the next time. Last, *check in with the implementer following the meeting to touch base about intervention fidelity and self-monitoring and answer any questions.* This follow-up will ensure that the implementer feels comfortable delivering the intervention and completing the self-monitoring tool after the meeting and that his or her questions have been answered. Confirm that the implementer knows how to contact you with any questions about the intervention or its implementation.

ADAPTATIONS TO SELF-MONITORING

The basic process of self-monitoring, in which an implementer rates his or her own intervention fidelity, is a relatively simple form of implementation support. In many cases, you will incorporate adaptations to increase the likelihood that the implementer will remember to self-monitor and continue to do so across time. There are four basic types of adaptations to self-monitoring (Table 8.1; Cooper et al., 2007). Antecedent-based tactics are design to make it more likely that the implementer will self-monitor by creating a prompt or reminder (e.g., setting a phone reminder, making a sign) or making self-monitoring easier to complete (e.g., clear, visually appealing forms embedded into current routines).

Adaptations that follow self-monitoring, such as self-evaluation, reinforcement, and performance feedback, are designed to increase the likelihood of self-monitoring in the future. Self-evaluation involves setting a goal about the frequency of self-monitoring or actual level of intervention fidelity. For instance, you might set a goal for the implementer that he or she self-monitors three times per week (i.e., frequency of self-monitoring), that particular intervention steps are delivered completely (i.e., actual level of intervention fidel-

TABLE 8.1. Adaptations to Self-Monitoring

Potential adaptations to self-monitoring	What does it involve?	When might it be applied?
Antecedent-based tactics	• Proactive efforts to make it more likely the implementer will self-monitor, including publically posting the self-monitoring form, providing prompts, setting a reminder to self-monitor, or embedding self-monitoring into regularly completed responsibilities.	• Whenever feasible; these simple, low-intensity strategies remind the implementer and make it easier for him or her to complete self-monitoring.
Self-evaluation	• Identify a self-monitoring and/or implementation goal (e.g., complete self-monitoring three times per week, adherence to 80% of intervention steps) to which the implementer can compare his or her behavior.	• When the implementer might benefit from some self-applied accountability to consistently self-monitor and increase his or her intervention fidelity, or if the implementer might need to work up to self-monitoring regularly (i.e., set stepwise goals)
Reinforcement	• Provide the implementer with reinforcement (e.g., small gift card, lunch, desired parking space, acknowledgment, coverage) once he or she has met a self-monitoring and/or intervention fidelity goal	• When the implementer might benefit from ongoing acknowledgment and reinforcement to maintain self-monitoring over time
Performance feedback	• Meeting to review intervention fidelity, learner outcomes, and self-monitoring data.	• When the implementer might benefit from external accountability to ensure consistent self-monitoring and improved intervention fidelity

ity), or that intervention fidelity is above 80% (i.e., actual level of intervention fidelity). When introducing self-monitoring, you might start by setting a goal for consistent completion of the self-monitoring tool, but once the implementer does this regularly, it would be appropriate to shift the goal to focus on intervention fidelity. Based on the data, determine an appropriate target (i.e., specific steps or the entire intervention) and criteria (e.g., level of adherence, level of quality). Reinforcement builds upon self-evaluation by including some sort of acknowledgment or reward when the goal is met. This can add salience to the goal and be motivating for some implementers. Performance feedback, described in Chapter 10, involves a brief meeting to review intervention fidelity, learner outcomes, and self-monitoring data; provide praise and feedback on implementation; and obtain the implementer's commitment to improve his or her implementation. Performance feedback can be delivered to target the implementer's completion of self-monitoring forms or the level of implementation, as indicated by the self-monitoring forms and intervention fidelity data. To identify the appropriate combination of adaptations, consider the suggestions in Table 8.1 as well as the implementer and the context.

Whatever combination of adaptations is added to self-monitoring, make sure to check the effectiveness of the entire self-monitoring plan. That is, evaluate any changes to intervention fidelity once the implementer begins engaging in self-monitoring. If improvement in the implementer's completion of the self-monitoring forms and/or intervention fidelity levels have not been observed after a period of time, it may be appropriate to reconsider which adaptations are being applied and either make modifications or additions. Also, as this strategy involves the implementer's engagement in behavior independently, make sure to regularly check in and be open to modifying the self-monitoring plan over time.

SUMMARY

Unlike other forms of implementation support described in this book, the focus of this strategy is a new activity in which the implementer will engage alongside the implementer of the intervention. To complete the self-monitoring, the implementer will systematically rate his or her delivery of some or all intervention steps. By simply attending to his or her implementation through self-monitoring, the implementer's intervention fidelity is likely to increase. During the self-monitoring session, the implementer will learn why and how to self-monitor, and together you will review and design a self-monitoring tool, consider potential adaptations, and discuss follow-up activities. Self-monitoring encourages the implementer to evaluate his or her own intervention fidelity independently; research suggests that self-monitoring is a feasible and effective form of implementation support (e.g., Belfiore et al., 2008; Simonsen et al., 2013).

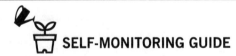

APPENDIX 8.1

Self-Monitoring Guide

Consultant: _____ Implementer: _____ Date: _____

Learner: _____ Intervention: _____ Start/End Time: _____

READINESS CHECKLIST

✓	**Have you . . .**
	1. Reviewed the intervention and current data?
☐	Familiarized yourself with the intervention plan?
☐	Reviewed the intervention fidelity data collection form?
☐	Reviewed the intervention goal and, using data, the learner's current progress?
☐	Evaluated intervention fidelity data?
	2. Prepared for self-monitoring?
☐	Read about self-monitoring?
☐	Created the first draft of the self-monitoring tool?
☐	Practiced dialogue, as needed, to be comfortable at the meeting?
	3. Identified session logistics?
☐	Scheduled the self-monitoring session?
☐	Reached out to the implementer?
☐	Brought self-monitoring materials to the session?

SELF-MONITORING GUIDE

Step 1: Explain the Purpose of the Session

- Provide an overview of self-monitoring.
- If available, highlight learner outcome data.
- Begin self-monitoring in an open, supportive manner.

Following is an example of what you might say to explain the purpose of this session.

> "Today, we're here to talk about the [*intervention*] and a plan for you to rate your own intervention fidelity. When people rate their own behavior, they naturally pay attention to it more, and it ends up increasing the desired behavior. To talk through this, we'll review the intervention and make a self-monitoring plan together."

(continued)

Step 2: Review the Intervention and Available Intervention Fidelity Data

- Describe the how and why of each intervention step.
- If available, highlight intervention fidelity data.

  "Let's start with the first step. To deliver it, you will [*describe how to deliver the intervention step*], which is important because it [*describe why the intervention step matters*]. Currently, it seems like [*describe intervention fidelity data*]."

Step 3: Review and Finalize the Self-Monitoring Tool

- Review the draft of the self-monitoring form and the potential rating options.
- Collaborate to finalize the self-monitoring tool.

  "Let's take a look at how you can track your intervention fidelity. When you're monitoring your implementation of this step, use [*describe the self-monitoring rating method*]. What do you think? Other options include [*describe other rating options*]."

Step 4: Practice Self-Monitoring

- Model how to self-monitor the intervention steps.
- Have the implementer practice completing the form.
- Provide positive yet corrective feedback.

  "If you delivered the intervention like [*explain intervention fidelity*], you would give yourself a [*explain the method of rating his or her self-monitoring*]. If you delivered the intervention like [*explain intervention fidelity*], what rating would you provide?"

Step 5: Decide Whether to Incorporate Any Self-Monitoring Adaptations

- Explain adaptations to the self-monitoring tool and the potential benefits.
- Decide if and which adaptations will be included.

(continued)

"There are a few different options with which to customize self-monitoring to include preparation and follow-up activities. Let's talk about if any of these might make sense to you going forward." [*Review adaptation options.*]

_____

_____

_____

Step 6: Make a Plan for Collecting Self-Monitoring Data

- Decide when and how often the implementer will self-monitor.
- Make a plan to calibrate self-monitoring ratings.

"Now that we have customized the self-monitoring, let's make a plan for our next steps. You implement the intervention [*indicate the frequency*], so you could self-monitor [*indicate the frequency*]. We should also make a plan to double-check the ratings to make sure that the form is clear and that you are comfortable completing it accurately."

_____

_____

_____

Step 7: Review the Meeting and Thank the Implementer

- Review the discussion and decisions made in the meeting.
- Thank the implementer and close the meeting.

"We discussed the [intervention] and made a plan for self-monitoring. It seems like we developed a plan for going forward. Any questions? [*Answer any questions.*] Thank you for meeting with me and remember that I'll be coming by soon to observe as you get started on self-monitoring."

_____

_____

_____

FOLLOW-UP CHECKLIST

✓	Have you . . .
☐	Reviewed session notes and completed the Fidelity Data Sheet for Self-Monitoring (Appendix 8.2) to ensure that the strategy was delivered as planned?
☐	Provided the agreed-upon version of the self-monitoring form and the Preparation Worksheet for Self-Monitoring (Appendix 8.3)?
☐	Calibrated the implementer's self-monitoring?
☐	Checked in with the implementer following the meeting to touch base about intervention fidelity and self-monitoring and to answer any questions?

Fidelity Data Sheet for Self-Monitoring

For each of the strategy steps, provide a rating of adherence (to what extent you covered each step), and of quality (how well you delivered each step) based on the following rubric.

Adherence	Quality
2 = All components of step delivered. 1 = Some components of step delivered. 0 = No components of step delivered.	2 = Step delivered in a smooth, natural manner, responsive to the implementer, and with appropriate nonverbal interaction. 1 = Step delivered with some aspects of quality. 0 = Step delivered without any aspects of quality.

Strategy Steps	Adherence	Quality
1. Explain the purpose of the session.		
2. Review the intervention and available intervention fidelity data.		
3. Review and finalize the self-monitoring tool.		
4. Practice self-monitoring.		
5. Decide whether to incorporate any self-monitoring adaptations.		
6. Make a plan for collecting self-monitoring data.		
7. Review the meeting and thank the implementer.		

First, sum each column:

              14   14

Next, divide by the number of steps to identify a percentage:

= _____%   = _____%

Preparation Worksheet for Self-Monitoring

Implementer: _____   Consultant: _____   Date: _____

Self-Monitoring Form: *Make sure the self-monitoring form meets the following criteria.*

✓ Includes all intervention steps or steps identified per intervention fidelity data.

✓ Has ratings for adherence, quality, and/or exposure.

✓ Is easy to understand, feasible to complete, and visually appealing.

Adaptations to Self-Monitoring: *Consider making adaptations to the self-monitoring form. Include details (e.g., goals, dates) below.*

Antecedent-based self-monitoring tactics (e.g., providing prompts):
Self-evaluation (i.e., compare self-monitoring to a goal):
Self-monitoring with reinforcement (i.e., receive a reward for meeting the goal):
Performance feedback with self-monitoring (i.e., meet to discuss data and self-monitoring):

Create Self-Monitoring Data Collection Plan: *Outline the plan for self-monitoring*

When will the implementer self-monitor? _____

_____

How often will the implementer self-monitor? _____

_____

Include date(s) for self-monitoring calibration: _____

_____

_____

CHAPTER 9

Motivational Interviewing

WHAT IS MOTIVATIONAL INTERVIEWING?

Motivational interviewing is a collaborative conversation guided by behavior change principles that strengthens an individual's—in this case, the implementer's—motivation and commitment to change (Box 9.1; Miller & Rollnick, 2013). In the context of motivational interviewing, ambivalence about changing any behavior is viewed as normal; the goal is to help people resolve their ambivalence in the direction of behavior change (not sustaining the status quo; in this case, low levels of intervention fidelity). You will use a collaborative, guiding conversational style designed to help implementers talk about their desire, ability, reasons, need, and/or commitment to change their intervention implementation behavior.

Your primary goal is to ask guiding questions such that the implementer talks about improving his or her intervention fidelity. You will achieve this by responding positively to such "change talk," while responding neutrally or not at all to talk about maintaining insufficient intervention fidelity (see Figure 9.1 on page 160 for examples of change talk). For example, you will provide praise, be encouraging, or ask for more information when an implementer talks about knowing the importance of intervention implementation, being confident in his or her ability to implement the intervention, or being ready to implement the intervention. If an implementer says, "I know implementing the intervention is important, but my afternoons are so busy, I keep forgetting," you would respond positively and solely to the statement that intervention implementation is important (i.e., "It's great we are both on the same page about how important implementing this intervention is to the learner's success"). Following a successful motivational implementation session, the implementer (not you!) will have provided the reasons to improve his or her intervention fidelity and, ideally, will have made a commitment to that change. Implementers will vary in how many motivational interviewing sessions they require to become committed to improving their levels of intervention fidelity. The amount of improvement needed for intervention fidelity to be sufficient, as well as the implementer's pace of change, may be key variables influencing the number of sessions needed.

BOX 9.1. MOTIVATIONAL INTERVIEWING SNAPSHOT

Who? Implementers who have demonstrated that they can deliver the intervention with sufficient intervention fidelity, but their current intervention fidelity (1) is variable across days, (2) has been high but is decreasing over time, or (3) is not occurring as frequently as it should.

What? Motivational interviewing occurs in a meeting in which you use a collaborative, guiding conversational style to help the implementer talk about his or her desire, ability, reasons, need, and/or commitment to improve his or her intervention delivery behavior.

Where? When? Complete motivational interviewing in a private space with just you and the implementer.

Why? Through motivational interviewing, you increase the implementer's statements about the importance and benefits of delivering the intervention with sufficient fidelity as well as his or her ability to do so. The more the implementer hears him- or herself talk about an ability to change, the more likely he or she is to commit to, and engage in, the delivery of intervention behaviors.

RESEARCH ON MOTIVATIONAL INTERVIEWING

There is considerable empirical evidence that provides compelling support for the idea that using motivational interviewing can increase a person's change talk, and that there is a relationship between the amount of change talk and actual behavior change (Frey, Sims, & Alvares, 2013; Miller & Rollnick, 2013). Motivational interviewing has been effectively applied to a wide variety of health conditions (e.g., increasing physical activity, decreasing alcohol use; Hettema, Steele, & Miller, 2005; O'Halloran, Shields, Blackstock, Wintle, & Taylor, 2016). Results suggest that motivational interviewing is effective as a stand-alone intervention or when used in combination with other strategies to support behavior change (e.g., goal setting, modeling, performance feedback; Draxten, Flattum, Fulkerson, 2016; Walker et al., 2017). Further, there are initial evaluations supporting the use of motivational interviewing as an effective approach to increasing intervention implementation in school- and community-based settings (Collier-Meek, Sanetti, et al., 2018; Hettema, Ernst, Williams, & Miller, 2014; Reinke, Lewis-Palmer, Merrell, 2008). The "elicit–provide–elicit" technique built into this chapter has been effectively used as a brief motivational interviewing approach to increase intervention implementation (Hettema et al., 2005). Importantly, research suggests that it is essential to follow the client's lead regarding when to engage in planning for change. Pushing such planning before the client is ready has resulted in decreased change talk and commitment to change (Hettema et al., 2005).

Desire to change
"I really want to implement this intervention because I know it is what Juan needs."
"I want all of my students to be ready for the third grade by the end of the year."

Ability to change
"I have implemented interventions like this in the past."
"It seems like I can fit this into my classroom routine."
"I am really organized, so I can keep track of all this."

Reasons to change
"If I can decrease the number of behavioral issues in the classroom, I will be able to teach them more and to have more fun."
"I know if I do this, her reading will improve and she will feel so much better about herself as a learner."
"This can help me get control of the classroom again; then I'll be able to have more fun with my students."

Need to change
"I have always loved teaching, but this has been a rough year; something has to change."
"Some of my students are not making the academic progress they need to make; decreasing the number of disruptions certainly might help them."
"I am just so exhausted at the end of the day, I can hardly do anything else."

Commitment to change
"I will try your suggestions; now I see how they can help my students."
"Tomorrow morning I am going to start by praising students who come in and start their writing prompt right away."
"I will make a poster of the behavioral expectations this weekend and fill it in with the kids on Monday during circle."

FIGURE 9.1. Types of change talk.

HOW DOES MOTIVATIONAL INTERVIEWING WORK?

Motivational interviewing is based on client-centered counseling principles and is rooted in social psychology (Miller & Rollnick, 2013). Its foundational idea is that how a person talks about change is directly related to his or her behavior. That is, the more a person talks about changing, the more likely he or she is to change. Alternatively, the more a person talks about reasons *not* to change, the less likely he or she to change. People learn about their own attitudes and beliefs by hearing themselves talk about them. Motivational interviewing is an approach that attempts to accelerate the change process by moving individuals out of ambivalence and toward change.

The motivational interviewing process empowers change talk through a guiding conversational style based on four fundamental processes (Miller & Rollnick, 2013). Using a guiding style (as opposed to a directing or following style; see Figure 9.2), you listen carefully, establish expertise when needed, evoke and explore change talk, ignore nonchange talk, and create a nonjudgmental working relationship. The four fundamental processes that facilitate a guiding style are (1) *engaging* the implementer in a working relationship, (2) *focusing* the conversation on intervention implementation, (3) *eliciting* the implementer's own motivations for change, and (4) *planning* the change (Miller & Rollnick, 2013). (Note: You can implement motivational interviewing without engaging in the fourth process, but the first three are necessary.) Across these processes, there are four core strategies used to

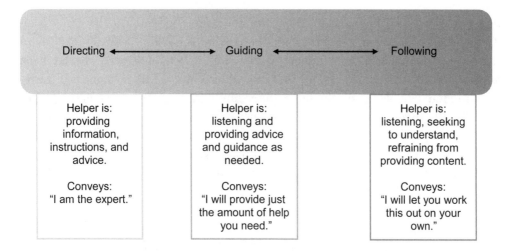

FIGURE 9.2. Types of communication styles.

guide individuals to engage in "change talk": open-ended questions, affirmations, reflections, and summaries, often shortened to the acronym *OARS* (Miller & Rollnick, 2013; see Figure 9.3). *Open-ended questions* are those that cannot be responded to with a "yes" or "no" answer. This type of question encourages the implementer to do most of the talking, and will allow you to learn about the implementer's experiences, feelings, thoughts, beliefs, and behaviors. *Affirmations* are statements that provide emotional support or encouragement and will help you build rapport and provide positive feedback for change-related talk. *Reflections* are statements in which you repeat, rephrase, or paraphrase the content and

Open-ended questions
   "How is the intervention going in your classroom?"
   "What concerns do you have about the learner?"
   "How do you hope I may be able to help you?"

Affirmations
   "You have thought a lot about this."
   "I can tell how much you care about your students."
   "I see how hard you are trying to get it all done."

Reflections
   "You are trying your best, but you can't seem to do it all."
   "You truly want what is best for your students."
   "You are frustrated by how slowly things are happening."

Summaries
   "OK, let me see if I have this right. You are feeling really stressed by
      the number of students in your class who need a lot of support from
      you. You care a lot about all of them, and want to help them all as
      much as you can, but you just can't see how you can fit it all in. At
      the same time, you know that if you stop and think carefully about
      it and are planful, you can do it because you have done it before."

FIGURE 9.3. Examples of OARS.

feeling of what the implementer has been communicating. Reflections allow you to demonstrate that you are listening carefully, and allow the implementer to "hear" his or her own words, feelings, and/or behaviors reflected back to him or her. *Summaries* are statements in which you attempt to concisely review what the implementer has been saying, to ensure that you and the implementer share the same understanding. Summary statements should start by indicating that you are attempting to summarize (e.g., "OK, let me see if I understand so far . . ."), should focus on change talk (e.g., " . . . you know you can handle this change to your morning routine . . ."), and should end with an invitation to the implementer to let you know if your summary is accurate (e.g., "Did I miss anything?"). (Chapter 11 provides a case study of applying motivational interviewing.)

WHAT IMPLEMENTERS WILL BENEFIT FROM MOTIVATIONAL INTERVIEWING?

Motivational interviewing will benefit implementers who have demonstrated that they can sufficiently implement the intervention (i.e., they have all the skills to implement the intervention), but their current intervention fidelity (1) is variable across days (e.g., full intervention fidelity one day, moderate intervention fidelity the next); (2) has been high but is decreasing over time; or (3) is not occurring as frequently as it should (e.g., supposed to deliver the intervention daily, but only delivering it 3 days per week). Motivational interviewing will not increase an implementer's skill or fluency with implementation. Thus, it is possible that an implementer who is both ambivalent about implementation and whose intervention fidelity data indicates some skill deficits (e.g., some intervention steps not delivered at all) may benefit from both motivational interviewing and a skill-building strategy (e.g., direct training).

GETTING READY FOR MOTIVATIONAL INTERVIEWING

Motivational interviewing is a conversation-based implementation support strategy that requires some preparation ahead of time to allow for a smooth and productive session with the implementer. Getting ready to deliver motivational interviewing involves three steps, outlined in Box 9.2 and described in the following sections. If you believe you need additional resources to support your use of motivational interviewing, consider the resources noted in Figure 9.4.

Step 1: Review the Intervention and Current Data

To prepare for motivational interviewing, review the intervention and current data. *Familiarize yourself with the intervention plan* so that you can fluently guide a conversation regarding the how-to and why of each intervention step, if needed. During the meeting, you will be focused on guiding the implementer to talk positively about implementing the intervention. As such, it is essential that you are very familiar with the intervention and,

---

BOX 9.2. Getting Ready to Deliver Motivational Interviewing

1. Review the intervention and current data.
   - Familiarize yourself with the intervention plan.
   - Review the intervention goal and, using data, the learner's current progress.
   - Evaluate intervention fidelity data.
2. Prepare for motivational interviewing.
   - Read about motivational interviewing.
   - Practice dialogue, as needed, to be comfortable at the meeting.
3. Identify session logistics.
   - Schedule the motivational interviewing session.
   - Reach out to the implementer.
   - Bring motivational interviewing materials to the session.

---

ideally, how it fits with the implementer's competing responsibilities, the physical environment, and other activities occurring in the implementation context. In addition, you will make a list of benefits that accrue from delivering the intervention with sufficient fidelity to facilitate your discussion with the implementer. Also, *review the intervention goal and the learner's progress data,* and *evaluate intervention fidelity data* to be comfortable describing current patterns in these data sources (e.g., level, trend, variability, relationship between data sources). Make graphs to illustrate this information and to guide your questioning with

Books
Miller, W. R., & Rollnick, S. (2013). *Motivational interviewing: Helping people change* (3rd ed.). New York: Guilford Press.
Reinke, W. M., Herman, K. C., & Sprick, R. (2011). *Motivational interviewing for effective classroom management: The classroom check-up.* New York: Guilford Press.
Rollnick, S., Kaplan, S. G., & Rutschman, R. (2016). *Motivational interviewing in schools: Conversations to improve behavior and learning.* New York: Guilford Press.
Rosengren, D. B. (2018). *Building motivational interviewing skills: A practitioner workbook* (2nd ed.). New York: Guilford Press.

Internet-Based Resources		
Organization or Agency	**Scope**	**Websites**
Motivational Interviewing Network of Trainers	Motivational interviewing trainings, resources, guides, and videos	*www.motivationalinterviewing.org*
Sobell, C. C., & Sobell, M. B. (2008). *Motivational interviewing strategies and techniques: Rationales and examples.*	A nine-page handout with the rationale and sample wording for numerous motivational interviewing strategies and techniques	*www.nova.edu/gsc/forms/mi_ rationale_techniques.pdf*
Substance Abuse and Mental Health Services Administration, Heath Resources and Services Administration, Center for Integrated Health Solutions	Resources and webinars on motivational interviewing	*www.integration.samhsa.gov/ clinical-practice/motivational-interviewing*

FIGURE 9.4. Books and Internet-based resources for motivational interviewing.

the implementer. Intervention steps that are being implemented well provide content for questions that are likely to elicit positive talk about implementation. Likewise, intervention steps that are being implemented inconsistently or not at all could elicit sustain talk, if asked about, and highlight opportunities to guide the conversation to positive change talk.

Step 2: Prepare for Motivational Interviewing

To be comfortable delivering this strategy, carefully *read about motivational interviewing,* and familiarize yourself with the strategy steps and talking points. Confirm your understanding of the purpose of the strategy and each of the steps. To *practice your dialogue,* review the Motivational Interviewing Guide (Appendix 9.1), intervention fidelity data, and intervention outcome data. It may also be helpful to create a "cheat sheet" of questions or types of questions that you might use during the session to ensure that you are using a guiding approach to the conversation, rather than a directive or following one. Similarly, be sure to review the OARS tools in Figure 9.3 and have some ready to use throughout your conversation with the implementer. This preparation will help you to maximize the strategy session and feel comfortable responding to the implementer.

Step 3: Identify Session Logistics

Once ready, it is necessary to plan the session logistics. To *schedule motivational interviewing,* determine when to hold the meeting. Plan to meet for approximately 30–45 minutes, although some motivational interviewing sessions may be shorter or longer. Although there may be more than one person implementing the intervention (e.g., paraprofessionals, school support professionals), motivational interviewing sessions should only include you and one implementer. Such a one-to-one session is necessary to fully engage with and respond to the implementer's unique perspective. Arrange where you will meet; you will need a quiet space that offers privacy for discussion and practice. Make sure time and location are feasible for the implementer. *Reach out to the implementer* ahead of the motivational interviewing session. Let the implementer know you will be discussing his or her delivery of the intervention and that you are very interested in getting his or her perspective on how things are going. Ask the implementer if there are any materials that might help him or her prepare for this conversation (e.g., written list of intervention steps, sample intervention materials, research, data). *Bring motivational interviewing materials to the session.* These materials include the Motivational Interviewing Guide (Appendix 9.1), two copies of the Planning for Change Worksheet (Appendix 9.2), the written intervention plan, a list of the benefits of intervention implementation, and graphs of intervention fidelity and learner outcome data.

MOTIVATIONAL INTERVIEWING STEP-BY-STEP

In using motivational interviewing in our context, you guide a conversation with the implementer about intervention implementation. The 14 steps of a motivational interviewing session and how they align with the four fundamental processes are listed in Box 9.3. The

---

BOX 9.3. Motivational Interviewing Steps and Processes

Engaging

1. Explain the purpose of the session.

Focusing

2. Elicit the implementer's perception of intervention implementation.
3. Summarize and validate the implementer's perceptions and reinforce change talk.
4. Review the implementation plan and intervention fidelity data.

Eliciting

5. Have implementer rate the importance of delivering the intervention as planned.
6. Summarize the rating of importance and elicit change talk.
7. Elicit the implementer's perspective on the benefits of implementing the intervention.
8. Provide a list of benefits of delivering the intervention with high fidelity.
9. Elicit the implementer's perspective on the benefits that increase the likelihood of delivering the intervention.
10. Have the implementer rate his or her confidence in his or her ability to deliver the intervention.
11. Summarize the rating of confidence and elicit change talk.
12. Determine what's next.

Planning

13. Engage the implementer in planning for change.
14. Review the meeting and thank the implementer.

Motivational Interviewing Guide (Appendix 9.1) includes the key objectives and sample language for each step, as well as space for recording implementer responses (focus on change talk and potential barriers). This guide can be copied and used for delivering this implementation support in your practice. A description of the steps in motivational interviewing, including key objectives and quick tips for delivery, are provided in the following sections.

Step 1: Explain the Purpose of the Session

• Provide an overview of motivational interviewing.
• Begin motivational interviewing in an open, supportive manner.

Describe the overall purpose of the motivational interviewing session so that the implementer understands what the meeting will entail and his or her role in it. For instance, you might say that you will be discussing implementation and getting the implementer's perspective on the intervention and its implementation. A key aspect of motivational interviewing is maintaining a nonjudgmental attitude. Create a supportive, nonjudgmental tone from the beginning by explaining that you want to know how the implementer is experiencing implementation so that you can work together to meet your collective goal of improving learner outcomes.

Step 2: Elicit the Implementer's Perception of Intervention Implementation

- Using an open-ended question, ask the implementer about how he or she thinks implementation has been going.

Ask the implementer to describe his or her perspective on how implementation has been going so far. Use open-ended questions to elicit the implementer's beliefs related to implementation (e.g., "How do you think your delivery of the intervention plan has been going?"). If the implementer provides brief or nondescriptive responses (e.g., "It's been fine"), continue asking open-ended questions that guide the implementer to provide more information about implementation (e.g., "What part of delivering the intervention is going the best for you?"; "What parts of the intervention does the learner react to the most positively?"; "Are there any parts of the intervention that you would like to deliver better?"). Note how the sample questions guide the implementer to engage in a positive response regarding the intervention. **How you word your open-ended questions can increase or decrease the likelihood of the implementer responding with change talk!**

Step 3: Summarize and Validate the Implementer's Perceptions and Reinforce Change Talk

- Summarize and validate the implementer's perceptions.
- Respond positively (verbally and nonverbally) to change talk.

Summarize the implementer's perceptions of the current implementation (e.g., "So, it seems like . . ."). As part of this step, validate the implementer's perceptions and feelings through empathic responses (e.g., "OK, so you know you want to use more of the positive response strategies, but it can be hard to remember to use them"). Remember, validating the implementer's perspective does not necessarily mean you agree with it; rather, you are acknowledging that it is the way he or she feels, and you are demonstrating your understanding. Additionally, emphasize and reinforce any change talk in the implementer's responses (e.g.,

---

Quick Tip 9.1. Managing Barriers during Motivational Interviewing

 When an implementer communicates aspects of delivering the intervention that are challenges, make a note of the potential barrier on your Motivational Interviewing Guide (Appendix 9.1). The barriers communicated by the implementer may provide information about additional supports or resources that are necessary to improve intervention fidelity. Be sure not to respond verbally to the challenges; rather, focus your reflections and summaries on change talk.

"You like the feeling of providing more praise to your students"). You may want to elicit more discussion related to the change talk as well (e.g., "How is your classroom different when you provide more praise?"). Summarize the implementer's responses and confirm that the summary was accurate (e.g., "Does that sound about right?"). If it was not accurate, repeat the summary process.

Step 4: Review the Implementation Plan and Intervention Fidelity Data

- Discuss the intervention plan and intervention fidelity data.
- Elicit the implementer's perspective on intervention fidelity data.
- Elicit change talk. ("What is/would be different when the intervention is implemented well?")

Discuss the status of implementation by reviewing the intervention implementation plan developed during implementation planning (Chapter 5, or the written intervention plan if you did not complete implementation planning) and graphed intervention fidelity data. Ask the implementer what he or she notices about the intervention fidelity data (e.g., "What do you see when you review these implementation data?"). Summarize and validate the implementer's response (e.g., "Yes, I agree, I see that some days are better than others") and elicit change talk as appropriate (e.g., "What is different on days that are better?"). For implementers who have a hard time interpreting the data or who respond ambivalently (e.g., "I don't really know"), provide your perspective (e.g., "What I see is that _____. What do you think?"). When expressing your perspective, focus on identifying intervention steps that the implementer is delivering with high fidelity and provide praise. Elicit the implementer's perspective about how things might be different if he or she demonstrated improved implementation (e.g., "How might things be different if you implemented the whole intervention [the intervention more often/the intervention for a longer period]?" or "How were things different when you did implement the intervention as planned?"). Summarize and validate the implementer's responses (e.g., "You believe that the learner might make better progress if you implemented the intervention consistently").

Step 5: Have the Implementer Rate the Importance of Delivering the Intervention as Planned

- Ask the implementer to rate the importance of delivering the intervention as planned on a 0–10 scale.

Ask the implementer to rate the importance of consistent, high-quality intervention implementation on a 0–10 scale. The typical question is, "On a scale from 0 to 10, with 0 being 'not at all important' and 10 being 'extremely important,' how important do you think it is for you to deliver _____ as we planned?" This rating will (1) inform you about how the implementer regards implementation and (2) provide an opening for a conversation about implementation.

Step 6: Summarize the Rating of Importance and Elicit Change Talk

- Provide a summary of the implementer's rating.
- Question why the rating was higher than another (lower) number.

Provide a brief summary of the implementer's rating (e.g., "A 3—OK, implementing this intervention is somewhat important to you"; "Wow, a 9! Implementing this intervention is very important to you!"). Then elicit change talk by asking a follow-up question about why his or her rating wasn't lower (e.g., "So, tell me, why are you at a 3 and not a zero?"; "Why are you an 8 and not a 5?"). The key here is to focus on why the implementer's rating was higher than another number. If you ask why their rating was lower than another number, you are likely to elicit talk about the challenges to implementation—which can be counterproductive in this approach. Instead, when you focus on why the implementer's rating was higher than another number, you are more likely to elicit change talk. It is rare that an implementer will provide a rating of zero, but if he or she does so, you can respond using an exaggerated reflection (e.g., "Whoa, a zero. OK, there is absolutely not a single thing in your life that is less important than implementing this intervention right now"). It is important that exaggerated reflections are delivered in a matter-of-fact voice, with no hint of joking or sarcasm. If the implementer admits that delivering the intervention is somewhat important, you might then ask the implementer to rate the importance of consistent, high-quality intervention implementation on a 0–10 scale again (i.e., repeat Step 5), and summarize his or her new rating (i.e., repeat Step 6). These types of reflections can help you determine how committed the implementer is to his or her rating.

Step 7: Elicit the Implementer's Perspective on the Benefits of Implementing the Intervention

- Ask the implementer about the benefits of implementing the intervention with high intervention fidelity.
- Respond positively (verbally and nonverbally) to change talk, while not responding to nonchange talk.

Regardless of the implementer's rating of the importance of intervention implementation, next ask the implementer about his or her perspective on the benefits of implementing the intervention. Your questioning in this step is especially important to the goal of engaging the implementer in talk about the positive aspects of consistent, high-quality intervention implementation. Remember, motivational interviewing is based on the theory that how a person talks about change is directly related to his or her behavior. That is, the more the implementer talks about the benefits of delivering the intervention with a high level of fidelity, the more likely he or she is to do so.

To ask an implementer about his or her perspective on the benefits of implementing the intervention, you might say, "What are some of the benefits of delivering [intervention name] in your [setting]?" This question focuses the conversation on the positive aspects of delivering the intervention with high fidelity. In his or her response, the implementer may acknowledge some benefits, but also convey some resistance. Respond differently to each type of statement. Reinforce all the benefits suggested by the implementer through your verbal (e.g., "Yes, I agree") and nonverbal (e.g., nodding head in agreement) responses, trying to elicit more discussion about intervention delivery from the implementer (e.g., "Tell me more about that"). Don't react verbally to statements of resistance (e.g., "Although I know doing the intervention is important, I just can't seem to fit it into my routine"); however, it may be beneficial to write down any barriers to intervention delivery that are suggested (e.g., lack of fit with routine).

Step 8: Provide a List of Benefits of Delivering the Intervention with High Fidelity

- Share the benefits of delivering the intervention with high intervention fidelity with the implementer.
- Focus on the benefits mentioned by the implementer.

Provide the previously developed list of benefits that accrue from delivering the intervention with sufficient intervention fidelity. As you talk through them, tie as many as you can to what the implementer just said (e.g., "Like you just mentioned, delivering the intervention consistently will enable the learner to improve her math skills more quickly; she might meet goal at the next benchmarking period!"; "You said that when you were delivering the intervention consistently, you had fewer behavioral issues to manage; increased engagement and decreased disruptive behavior are major benefits of implementing this intervention").

Step 9: Elicit the Implementer's Perspective on the Benefits That Increase the Likelihood of Delivering the Intervention

- Ask the implementer what benefits stand out to him or her.
- Reinforce change talk.
- Elicit more talk about the benefits of delivering the intervention with high fidelity.

Having reviewed the benefits of intervention implementation, ask the implementer what benefits stood out the most to him or her or would be most likely to lead him or her to implement the intervention ("You've mentioned quite a few benefits to implementing this intervention; which ones strike you as important and relevant?"). Continue to reinforce all change talk through your verbal (e.g., "Yes, that is an important benefit") and nonverbal (e.g., nodding head in agreement) responses. Try to elicit more talk about the behaviors in which the implementer could engage to experience the benefits of delivering the intervention with high fidelity that he or she just identified as important and relevant (e.g., if the implementer identifies increased on-task student behavior as a benefit that could lead him or her to implement the intervention, you might say, "Tell me more about what you can do to help students demonstrate more on-task behaviors").

Summarize and validate the implementer's responses, highlighting the benefits of intervention implementation and the implementation behaviors in which the implementer has said he or she could engage (e.g., "[List benefits] are benefits of implementing this intervention that really stand out to you. To reap those benefits, you believe you can [insert list of implementation behaviors]. Did I get that right?").

Step 10: Have the Implementer Rate His or Her Confidence in His or Her Ability to Deliver the Intervention

- Ask the implementer to rate his or her confidence in his or her ability to deliver the intervention on a 0–10 scale.

The implementer has listed not only some benefits of delivering the intervention with high fidelity, but also some behaviors that are necessary to deliver the intervention. Ask the implementer to rate his or her confidence in his or her ability to demonstrate these intervention delivery behaviors on a 0–10 scale. The typical question, "On a scale from 0 to 10, with 0 being 'not at all confident' and 10 being 'extremely confident,' how confident are you that if you decided to [list behaviors related to delivering the intervention with high fidelity] consistently, you could do it?"

   This rating will inform your discernment of how close the implementer is to being ready for change. Remember that it is not enough to recognize the importance of the intervention to initiate change in how well the implementer delivers an intervention; in addition, the implementer needs to *believe* that he or she can do it. If an implementer's rating is somewhat low, it will be especially important to consider if another implementation support strategy may be needed to increase his or her confidence. For example, a skill-building strategy may increase the implementer's confidence in his or her ability to deliver each intervention step as planned, or a performance-building strategy may increase the implementer's confidence in his or her ability to consistently deliver the intervention with high fidelity.

Step 11: Summarize the Rating of Confidence and Elicit Change Talk

- Provide a summary of the implementer's rating.
- Question why the rating was higher than another (lower) number.

Provide a brief summary of the implementer's rating (e.g., "A 4—you are somewhat confident you can implement this intervention"; "A 7—OK, you are pretty confident!"; "Wow, a 9! You are really confident that you can do this!"). Then elicit change talk by asking a follow-up question about why the implementer's rating wasn't lower (e.g., "So, tell me, why are you at a 4 and not a zero?"; "Why are you a 7 and not a 5?"). The key here is to focus on why the implementer's rating was higher than another number. If you ask why the implementer's rating was lower than another number, you are likely to elicit talk about barriers to implementation—which can be counterproductive in this approach. Instead, when you focus on why the implementer's rating was higher than another number, you are more likely to elicit change talk. It is rare that an implementer will provide a rating of zero, but if they do, you can respond using an exaggerated reflection (e.g., "Whoa, a zero. You are not at all confident that you could deliver even a tiny little part of this intervention to benefit the learner right now"). As noted above, it is important that exaggerated reflections are delivered in a matter-of-fact voice, with no hint of joking or sarcasm. If the implementer admits that he or she is somewhat confident in his or her ability to deliver the intervention with a high level of fidelity, you might ask the implementer to rate his or her confidence in his or her ability to deliver the intervention on a 0–10 scale again (i.e., repeat Step 5), and then summarize their new rating (i.e., repeat Step 6). These types of reflections can help you determine how committed the implementer is to his or her rating.

Step 12: Determine What's Next

- Briefly summarize the implementer's change talk throughout the session.
- Ask the implementer a key question about what comes next.

At this point, you have engaged the implementer in a supportive working relationship, focused the discussion on intervention implementation, and elicited the implementer's own reasons for increasing intervention implementation. The last part of motivational interviewing is planning, which occurs when the implementer's motivation indicates that he or she is ready to shift from talking about *why he or she should change* to *how he or she will* change.

There isn't any hard-and-fast criterion with which to determine when someone is at this point. In general, if the implementer has a (1) moderate-to-high level of confidence about delivering the intervention, (2) has started engaging in more spontaneous change talk, or (3) has decreased the amount of ambivalence or resistance to delivering the intervention in his or her talk about intervention delivery across the session, it may be a sign that the implementer is ready to plan how to improve his or her intervention implementation. The only way to know for sure, however, is to ask.

First, summarize the implementer's change talk that has been expressed throughout the session. Do not editorialize; simply reflect back the motivations for implementing the intervention that the implementer has already identified for you. Hearing all the motivations together at once can be a powerful experience.

Second, ask a short and simple question about what's next; there are lots of ways this key question can be phrased (see Figure 9.5). This question is not asking for commitment; it's phrasing should not put pressure on the implementer. The summarization and key question together should convey, "Here are the motivations you identified for delivering the intervention consistently and completely. It's in your hands what, if anything, you choose to do. What do you think?"

If the implementer's response suggests that he or she is at all ready to start engaging in any changes toward increased intervention implementation, move to Step 13. If the implementer does not seem ready to plan changes (e.g., responses to the key question indicate that the implementer wants to think about the intervention more), then summarize and validate those responses, skip Step 13, and recommend that you and the implementer meet again to continue discussing implementation. In the next session, you may start by reviewing Step 5 (e.g., "Last time we met, you rated the importance of implementing the intervention X. Does that still sound about right?") and by continuing to focus on eliciting change

> - "So, where does all this leave you?"
> - "What are you thinking about intervention implementation at this point?"
> - "I wonder what you might decide to do about this intervention."
> - "After all we have discussed, what do you think you might do?"
> - "So, what's next?"
> - "What are you going to do from here?"
> - "Tell me what you think the next step is."
> - "What's our plan from here?"

FIGURE 9.5. Examples of key questions.

talk. Although it may be tempting, pushing the implementer to engage in change planning before he or she is ready will likely backfire.

Step 13: Engage the Implementer in Planning for Change

- Ask the implementer if he or she is ready to plan for change.
- Complete the Planning for Change Worksheet (Appendix 9.2) with the implementer.

For implementers whose response to the key question indicate that they are ready to engage in some level of behavior change related to intervention implementation (even if it is a small change!), ask if they are interested in coming up with a plan for that change (e.g., "It sounds like you really want to implement more of this plan! Shall we talk about the plan for moving forward?"). Give the implementer a copy of the Planning for Change Worksheet (Appendix 9.2; you should have your own copy as well). Tell the implementer that this worksheet will help him or her plan those aspects of their intervention delivery that he or she wants to change, identify why he or she wants to change those aspects, how to go about it, what support is needed, how both of you will know if the change is working, and what both of you will do if no change occurs. Talk the implementer through completion of each step of the Planning for Change Worksheet (Appendix 9.2), instructing the implementer to write his or her responses on his or her worksheet, while you write your responses on your worksheet. Continue to reinforce the implementer's change talk. Even if the implementer only chooses to improve a small number of intervention delivery behaviors (as opposed to all of them, which you might have been hoping for), remember it is a step in the right direction! Pay careful attention to the "Ways other people can help me" step; it is important to advocate for or facilitate the implementer's obtaining the help requested. It is possible that the implementer's responses at this point may indicate a need for additional resources, training, or performance support. If so, consider whether the implementer may benefit from a skill- or performance-building implementation strategy. For example, if obtaining resources is a concern, implementation planning, in which you consider the resources needed per intervention step, could be a good next step. Alternatively, if being accountable for consistency is a concern, performance feedback, in which you provide regular feedback on intervention fidelity, could be a good next step.

Step 14: Review the Meeting and Thank the Implementer

- Review the meeting discussion and decisions.
- Thank the implementer and close the meeting.

Close the motivational interviewing session by providing a summary of the meeting. In particular, highlight the discussions regarding the importance of intervention fidelity, the implementer's motivations for implementing the intervention, and the specific steps the implementer will take to improve his or her intervention implementation. In doing so, you provide a final opportunity to ensure that you and the implementer agree on the central aspects of the meeting and that you are both clear about the next steps needed to facilitate increased levels of intervention fidelity. End the meeting positively by thanking the implementer for engaging in the discussion about the intervention and encouraging him or her to be in touch with you if implementation issues arise.

FOLLOW-UP AFTER MOTIVATIONAL INTERVIEWING

To cement the discussion and progress made during motivational interviewing, we suggest that you engage in some activities after the session. Follow-up after motivational interviewing involves three steps, outlined in Box 9.4 and described in the next paragraph.

Review session notes to ensure that the strategy was delivered as planned. To do so, check the Motivational Interviewing Guide (Appendix 9.1) and complete a self-assessment using the Fidelity Data Sheet for Motivational Interviewing (Appendix 9.3) to see if you addressed each of the strategy steps. If you missed any steps, follow up with the implementer. It is important to make sure that the strategies were delivered as planned so that they have the most likelihood of impacting the implementer. If needed, *update the intervention plan and/or the implementation plan.* If any changes were made during motivational interviewing, especially during completion of the Planning for Change Worksheet (Appendix 9.2), update all written materials to reflect those changes. Share the updated materials with the implementer as soon as possible. Last, *check in with implementer following the meeting to touch base about implementation and answer any questions.* This follow-up will ensure that the implementer feels comfortable delivering the intervention after the meeting and that his or her questions have been answered. If needed, schedule another session with the implementer to explore further increasing his or her implementation fidelity, if further

---

BOX 9.4. Motivational Interviewing Follow-Up Steps

1. Review session notes to ensure that the strategy was delivered as planned.
2. Update the intervention plan and/or the implementation plan, as needed.
3. Check in with the implementer following the meeting to touch base about intervention fidelity and answer any questions.

behavioral change is needed. Confirm that the implementer knows how to contact you with any questions about the intervention or its implementation.

SUMMARY

Motivational interviewing is a collaborative conversational approach to discussing behavior change that increases the implementer's motivation for and commitment to intervention implementation. Motivational interviewing involves four processes: (1) *engaging* the implementer in a working relationship, (2) *focusing* the conversation on intervention implementation, (3) *eliciting* the client's motivation for change, and (4) *planning* the change. You use OARS (open-ended questions, affirmations, reflections, and summaries) and selectively reinforce the implementer's verbalizations that represent "change talk" (i.e., improved intervention implementation). When the implementer conveys increased motivation for and confidence in his or her ability to implement the intervention, he or she may be ready to engage in planning for change. When he or she is ready to plan, you guide the implementer through the development of a plan that outlines which aspects of intervention implementation he or she wants to change and identifies why he or she wants to change those aspects, how to go about it, what support is needed, how both of you will know if the change is working, and what both of you will do if no change occurs. After the motivational interviewing session, it may be clear that another session is needed to continue the momentum toward planning for change, or you will have completed the planning for change and the implementer will have a clear strategy with which to improve his or her implementation behavior.

Motivational Interviewing Guide

Consultant: _____   Implementer: _____   Date: _____

Learner: _____   Intervention: _____   Start/End Time: _____

READINESS CHECKLIST

✓	**Have you . . .**
	1. Reviewed the intervention and current data?
☐	Familiarized yourself with the intervention plan?
☐	Reviewed the intervention goal and, using data, the learner's current progress?
☐	Evaluated intervention fidelity data?
	2. Prepared for motivational interviewing?
☐	Read about motivational interviewing?
☐	Practiced dialogue, as needed, to be comfortable at the meeting?
	3. Identified session logistics?
☐	Scheduled the motivational interviewing session?
☐	Reached out to the implementer?
☐	Brought motivational interviewing materials to the session?

MOTIVATIONAL INTERVIEWING GUIDE

Step 1: Explain the Purpose of the Session

- Provide an overview of motivational interviewing.
- Begin motivational interviewing in an open, supportive manner.

Following is an example of what you might say to explain the purpose of this session.

"Thanks so much for taking the time to meet with me today. I wanted to talk a bit about how delivering [*intervention name*] for [*learner*] is going. Learning about your thoughts on the [*intervention name*] and how it's going so far is really important so we can meet our goal of helping [*learner*] meet his [*her*] goals."

_____

_____

_____

(continued)

Step 2: Elicit the Implementer's Perception of Intervention Implementation

- Using an open-ended question, ask the implementer about how he or she thinks implementation has been going.

    "How do you think your delivery of the intervention plan has been going?"

_____

_____

_____

Step 3: Summarize and Validate the Implementer's Perceptions and Reinforce Change Talk

- Summarize and validate the implementer's perspective.
- Respond positively (verbally and nonverbally) to change talk.

    "So, it seems like you agree that this intervention will help [*learner*], but you are finding it challenging to deliver some parts of it the way we talked about. You can see that she [*he*] really responds to specific praise when you provide it, and you like the way it feels to be pointing out what students are doing well. Does that sound about right?"

_____

_____

_____

Step 4: Review the Implementation Plan and Intervention Fidelity Data

- Discuss the intervention plan and intervention fidelity data.
- Elicit the implementer's perspective on intervention fidelity data.
- Elicit change talk ("What is/would be different when the intervention is implemented well?")

    "Here's the intervention plan we developed [*show plan*]. As you recall, we included [*discuss steps or strategies*]. Let's look at the information I have on how it has been going in your classroom [*show intervention fidelity data*]. What do you notice when you look at these data? Yes, I agree that some days are better than others. What is different on days that are better? How might things be different if more days were better?"

_____

_____

_____

Step 5: Have the Implementer Rate the Importance of Delivering the Intervention as Planned

- Ask the implementer to rate the importance of delivering the intervention as planned on a 0–10 scale.

    "On a scale from 0 to 10, with 0 being 'not at all important' and 10 being 'extremely important,' how important do you think it is for you to deliver [*intervention name*] as we planned?"

(continued)

_____

_____

_____

Step 6: Summarize the Rating of Importance and Elicit Change Talk

- Provide a summary of the implementer's rating.
- Question why the rating was higher than another (lower) number.

> "A [*insert rating number*], OK. So implementing this intervention is [*somewhat/very*] important to you. Why are you a [*insert rating number*] and not a [*insert number lower than rating*]?"

_____

_____

_____

Step 7: Elicit the Implementer's Perspective on the Benefits of Implementing the Intervention

- Ask the implementer about the benefits of implementing the intervention with high intervention fidelity.
- Respond positively (verbally and nonverbally) to change talk, while not responding to nonchange talk.

> "What are some of the benefits of delivering [*intervention name*] in your [*setting*]? [*Respond to change talk with statements such as:*] "Yes, I agree" or "Tell me more about that."

_____

_____

_____

Step 8: Provide a List of Benefits of Delivering the Intervention with High Fidelity

- Share the benefits of delivering the intervention with high intervention fidelity with the implementer.
- Focus on the benefits mentioned by the implementer.

> "There are numerous benefits that come from delivering this intervention with high fidelity. Like you just mentioned, [*highlight benefits mentioned by implementer that are on your list*]."

_____

_____

_____

Step 9: Elicit the Implementer's Perspective on the Benefits That Increase the Likelihood of Delivering the Intervention

- Ask the implementer what benefits stand out to him or her.
- Reinforce change talk.
- Elicit more talk about the benefits of delivering the intervention with high fidelity.

(continued)

"You've mentioned quite a few benefits that would come from implementing this intervention. Which ones strike you as important and relevant? [*After the implementer's response, follow up with questions about behaviors in which the implementer can engage to experience the benefit:*] Tell me more about what you can do to [*benefit*]."

_____

_____

_____

Step 10: Have the Implementer Rate His or Her Confidence in His or Her Ability to Deliver the Intervention

- Ask the implementer to rate his or her confidence in his or her ability to deliver the intervention on a 0–10 scale.

"On a scale of from 0 to 10, with 0 being 'not at all confident' and 10 being 'extremely confident,' how confident are you that if you decided to [*behaviors related to delivering the intervention with high fidelity*] consistently, you could do it?"

_____

_____

_____

Step 11: Summarize the Rating of Confidence and Elicit Change Talk

- Provide a summary of the implementer's rating.
- Question why the rating was higher than another (lower) number.

"A [*insert rating number*], OK. You are [*somewhat/very*] confident in your ability to deliver this intervention. Why are you a [*insert rating number*] and not a [*insert number lower than rating*]?"

_____

_____

_____

Step 12: Determine What's Next

- Briefly summarize the client's change talk throughout the session.
- Ask the implementer a key question about what's next.

"Throughout our conversation today, you have mentioned [*summarize change talk here*]. At this point, what are you thinking about intervention implementation?"

If implementer seems ready for change, move to the next step. If the implementer does not seem ready for change, say:

"It seems like we should meet again to figure out how we can move forward to help [*learner*] meet his [*her*] goal."

(continued)

_____

_____

_____

Step 13: Engage the Implementer in Planning for Change

- Ask the implementer if he or she is ready to plan for change.
- Complete the Planning for Change Worksheet (Appendix 9.2) with the implementer.

> "It sounds like you really want to implement more of this plan! Shall we talk about a plan for moving forward? [*If you get a positive response:*] OK, great! Let's take a look at this Planning for Change Worksheet [*Appendix 9.2*] that will help us make sure we cover all the bases as we move forward. [*Talk through worksheet with implementer.*]
>
> "[*If you get an ambivalent or negative response:*] You aren't quite ready to move forward with next steps yet, and that's OK! Let's set up a time to meet again and figure out how we can move forward to help [*learner*] meet her [*his*] goal."

_____

_____

_____

Step 14: Review the Meeting and Thank the Implementer

- Review the meeting discussion and decisions.
- Thank the implementer and close the meeting.

> "We have made a plan for the next steps [*insert any specifics from Planning for Change Worksheet*]. Do you have any questions about what we've covered? [*Answer any questions.*] Thank you for taking the time to talk about how this intervention is proceeding."

_____

_____

_____

FOLLOW-UP CHECKLIST

✓	Have you . . .
☐	1. Reviewed the session notes to ensure that the strategy was delivered as planned?
☐	2. Updated the intervention plan and/or the implementation plan, as needed?
☐	3. Checked in with the implementer following the meeting to touch base about intervention fidelity and answer any questions?

Planning for Change Worksheet

The changes I want to make (or continue making) are:
The reasons why I want to make these changes are:
The steps I plan to take in changing are:
The ways other people can help me change are:
I will know if my plan is working if:
Some things that could interfere with my plan are:
What I will do if the plan isn't working:

Fidelity Data Sheet for Motivational Interviewing

For each of the strategy steps, provide a rating of adherence (to what extent you covered each step) and of quality (how well you delivered each step) based on the following rubric.

Adherence	Quality
2 = All components of step delivered. 1 = Some components of step delivered. 0 = No components of step delivered.	2 = Step delivered in a smooth, natural manner, responsive to the implementer, and with appropriate nonverbal interaction. 1 = Step delivered with some aspects of quality. 0 = Step delivered without any aspects of quality.

Strategy Steps	Adherence	Quality
1. Explain the purpose of the session.		
2. Elicit the implementer's perception of intervention implementation.		
3. Summarize and validate the implementer's perceptions and reinforce change talk.		
4. Review the implementation plan and intervention fidelity data.		
5. Have the implementer rate the importance of delivering the intervention as planned.		
6. Summarize the rating of importance and elicit change talk		
7. Elicit the implementer's perspective on the benefits of implementing the intervention.		
8. Provide a list of benefits of delivering the intervention with high fidelity.		
9. Elicit the implementer's perspective on the benefits that increase the likelihood of delivering the intervention.		
10. Have the implementer rate his or her confidence in his or her ability to deliver the intervention.		
11. Summarize the rating of confidence and elicit change talk.		

(continued)

Strategy Steps	Adherence	Quality
12. Determine what's next.		
13. Engage the implementer in planning for change.		
14. Review the meeting and thank the implementer.		

First, sum each column:

                               28   28

Next, divide by number of steps to identify a percentage:

       = _____%   = _____%

CHAPTER 10

Performance Feedback

WHAT IS PERFORMANCE FEEDBACK?

Performance feedback is a form of implementation support that involves meeting with an implementer to review and discuss intervention fidelity data, including what is going well (i.e., intervention steps consistently implemented) and what is challenging (i.e., intervention steps inconsistently delivered; see Box 10.1). A graph of intervention fidelity data can be helpful to supplement this conversation and illustrate the current pattern of implementa-

---

BOX 10.1. Performance Feedback Snapshot

Who? Implementers who continue to struggle after other, less intensive implementation supports have been provided. Implementers who demonstrate inconsistent delivery of a high-intensity student intervention.

What? A brief meeting to review intervention fidelity data, discuss intervention fidelity strengths, review challenging intervention steps, and recommit to ongoing intervention delivery.

Where? When? Deliver it in 5–15 minutes on an ongoing (e.g., weekly) or as-needed basis in a private meeting space.

Why? It includes (1) praise for intervention steps delivered consistently to encourage implementers' intervention fidelity, and (2) reminders about accountability and challenging steps to provide practice.

---

tion. During this meeting, you may work with the teacher to reteach and/or problem-solve the inconsistently implemented intervention steps. In many cases, the learner's progress is also reviewed at this meeting, highlighting the link between implementation and learner outcomes. Other components, such as goal setting and self-monitoring, are sometimes incorporated into performance feedback, providing options to customize this strategy to fit the implementer and the context.

RESEARCH ON PERFORMANCE FEEDBACK

Performance feedback is a widely researched implementation support strategy. It was adapted from research and practice in industrial/organizational psychology for school-based practice in the mid-1990s by Noell and colleagues (e.g., Noell et al., 1997). Its effectiveness has been evaluated across individual, small group, and class-wide interventions to support learners with and without disabilities and with implementers such as general and special education teachers, paraprofessionals, and school teams (Fallon et al., 2015). Results of systematic reviews and meta-analyses, wherein multiple studies are evaluated together to identify effectiveness, indicate performance feedback consistently improves implementers' intervention fidelity (Fallon et al., 2015; Noell et al., 2014; Solomon et al., 2012). Performance feedback with visual and graphic feedback has been shown to have moderate effects on teachers' fidelity for classroom-based interventions, with a corresponding impact on learner outcomes (Solomon et al., 2012). Performance feedback has been shown to be most effective when delivered quickly following intervention delivery (as opposed to weekly), although study designs may have contributed to these findings. Meta-analysis results indicate that delivering the essential components of performance feedback resulted in a large effect, and performance feedback with Negative Reinforcement and performance feedback with Modeling or Role Play also resulted high levels of intervention fidelity (Noell et al., 2014). Results of a systematic review that applied What Works Clearinghouse Standards, suggested that performance feedback is an evidence-based practice (Fallon et al., 2015).

HOW DOES PERFORMANCE FEEDBACK WORK?

Performance feedback has been widely researched and is considered an effective form of implementation support (Noell & Gansle, 2013). It is based on behavioral theory and involves providing praise and positive feedback for steps that are consistently implemented. This praise, presumed to act as positive reinforcement, is thought to increase the likelihood that the implementer will continue to deliver these intervention steps consistently in the future. In addition, performance feedback includes discussion, reminders, and possibly practice of intervention steps that have not been consistently implemented. This process provides an opportunity for the implementer to relearn the intervention steps, for you to answer questions, and for you and the implementer to collaboratively problem-solve how to deliver these steps, while also providing accountability for delivering these steps consistently. This process ensures that the implementer is prepared for implementation and knows that you will follow up on his or her intervention fidelity.

WHAT IMPLEMENTERS WILL BENEFIT FROM PERFORMANCE FEEDBACK?

Although it can be used across a wide range of implementers, interventions, and situations, performance feedback is recommended for implementers who continue to struggle to deliver an intervention after receiving other, less intensive forms of implementation supports. Performance feedback is also appropriate as a first step to help an implementer who is struggling to deliver a high-intensity learner intervention (e.g., behavior support plan for a learner who is demonstrating dangerous behaviors, intensive academic intervention for a learner who is several grade levels behind). Why might performance feedback be particularly suited for these implementers? Although performance feedback meetings are usually relatively brief, with most lasting only 5–15 minutes, they are designed to be delivered on an ongoing basis. That is, consultants should be prepared to deliver performance feedback several times on a daily, weekly, or as-needed basis (i.e., when intervention fidelity drops). Thus, for most situations, it makes sense to begin with a proactive, one-time implementation support, such as implementation planning or self-monitoring, before engaging in performance feedback. For those situations that are high intensity, the strong evidence base for performance feedback suggests that it should be utilized when it is critical to rapidly improve intervention fidelity.

GETTING READY FOR PERFORMANCE FEEDBACK

Performance feedback involves a brief, conversation-based implementation support strategy that requires minimal preparation. However, taking the time to complete the necessary preparation steps will help the meeting go smoothly. Getting ready to deliver performance feedback involves three steps, outlined in Box 10.2 and described below.

Step 1: Review the Intervention and Current Data

To prepare for performance feedback, review the intervention and current data. *Familiarize yourself with the intervention plan* so that you are able to fluently describe the how-to and why of each intervention step as well as model and problem-solve delivering these steps with intervention fidelity. During the meeting, the implementer will refer to your expertise on the intervention and its implementation; be prepared to serve in this role. If not already completed, break the intervention into components (see Chapter 5). Also, *review the intervention goal and learner's progress* and *review intervention fidelity data* to be comfortable describing current patterns in these data sources (e.g., level, trend, variability, relationship between data sources). If possible, make graphs to illustrate this information, which can be used during the performance feedback session (see Chapter 3).

BOX 10.2. Getting Ready to Deliver Performance Feedback

1. Review the intervention and current data.
   - Familiarize yourself with the intervention plan.
   - Review the intervention goal and, using data, the learner's current progress.
   - Evaluate the intervention fidelity data.
2. Prepare to provide performance feedback.
   - Read about performance feedback.
   - Practice dialogue, as needed, to be comfortable at the meeting.
3. Identify session logistics.
   - Schedule the performance feedback session.
   - Reach out to the implementer.
   - Bring performance feedback materials to the session.

Step 2: Prepare to Provide Performance Feedback

To be comfortable delivering this strategy, carefully *read about performance feedback* and decide which components are appropriate to include, based on the context (see "Adaptations to Performance Feedback" on p. 194). Once the components have been identified, familiarize yourself with the strategy steps and talking points. Confirm your understanding of the purpose of the strategy and each of the steps. Prepare any necessary information or materials (e.g., graphs, reports, written intervention plan, research). To *practice your dialogue,* review the Performance Feedback Guide (see Appendix 10.1 at the end of this chapter), intervention fidelity data, and intervention outcome data. This preparation will help you to maximize the strategy session and feel comfortable addressing the individual implementer's concerns and needs. It may be helpful to (1) organize the intervention into a written list of teachable steps for the purpose of demonstration and practice, (2) identify target steps for practice based on implementation data, or (3) brainstorm potential scenarios to use for practicing the target steps.

Step 3: Identify Session Logistics

Once ready, it is necessary to plan the session logistics. To *schedule a meeting for performance feedback,* determine how long the meeting will last, when to hold the meeting, and how many sessions are needed to complete the strategy. Plan to meet for approximately 15 minutes, although some performance feedback sessions may be shorter or longer. Decide who will be involved (e.g., primary implementer, potential collaborators). In some cases, there is more than one person implementing the intervention (e.g., paraprofessionals, school support professionals) or other stakeholders (e.g., case worker, parent), who may be interested in attending. Arrange where you will meet. You will need a quiet space that offers privacy for discussion and practice. Make sure that time and location are feasible for the implementer. *Reach out to the implementer* ahead of the performance feedback session. If you think it would be helpful for the implementer to review any materials prior to the strategy meeting, provide those in advance (e.g., written list of intervention steps, sample intervention materials, research, data). *Bring the performance feedback materials* to the session. These materials include the Performance Feedback Guide (Appendix 10.1), the written intervention plan, and graphs of intervention fidelity and learner outcome data.

PERFORMANCE FEEDBACK STEP-BY-STEP

When providing performance feedback, you review and discuss the intervention with the implementer. The eight steps of a typical performance feedback session are listed in Box 10.3. The Performance Feedback Guide (see Appendix 10.1) includes the key objectives and sample language for each step, as well as space for recording the implementer's responses. This guide can be copied and used for delivering this implementation support in your practice. A description of the steps involved in giving performance feedback, including key objectives and quick tips for delivery, are provided in the following sections.

Step 1: Explain the Purpose of the Session

- Provide an overview of performance feedback.
- Begin providing performance feedback in an open, supportive manner.

Orient the implementer to performance feedback by providing an overview of the brief meeting session. Explain that, together, you and the implementer will talk about intervention fidelity and learner outcomes, consider the data, and brainstorm ways to support consistent delivery of the intervention. In doing so, you will start the performance feedback session in an open, collaborative, and supportive manner. Although you may highlight areas of improvement for the implementer, this meeting is not meant to be critical in nature. Rather, this meeting is successful when it is presented as an opportunity to look at a snapshot of current intervention fidelity data and learner outcomes, and to facilitate practice and problem solving in a supportive manner to improve ongoing intervention fidelity.

BOX 10.3. Performance Feedback Steps

1. Explain the purpose of the session.
2. Ask the implementer about intervention fidelity.
3. Ask the implementer about learner progress.
4. Review intervention fidelity data.
5. Review learner outcome data and highlight progress toward intervention goal.
6. Review and practice inconsistently delivered intervention steps.
7. Problem-solve how to improve progress toward the intervention fidelity goal and obtain the implementer's commitment to the plan.
8. Review the meeting and thank the implementer.

Step 2: Ask the Implementer about Intervention Fidelity

- Elicit the implementer's perspective on intervention fidelity.
- Summarize and validate the implementer's perspective.

Ask the implementer for his or her perspective on how intervention delivery has been progressing, highlighting your understanding that intervention fidelity isn't always easy, and that you want to help the implementer achieve successful implementation. Opening in this manner provides an opportunity for the implementer to reflect on what has been going well and what has been difficult. Further, eliciting the implementer's perspective will demonstrate your interest in his or her experiences and will help the interaction to feel collaborative, rather than evaluative. The implementer may ask questions about the intervention at this time. Answer to the best of your knowledge, but also feel comfortable telling the implementer that you will discuss specific issues or questions later (e.g., reviewing specifics of particular intervention steps, if appropriate). As the implementer shares his or her perspective, summarize and validate what the implementer has said. That is, use your own wording to restate what the implementer has said and acknowledge, in a supportive manner, the implementer's perspective. It will be helpful to refer back to the implementer's views in later steps involving performance feedback.

Step 3: Ask the Implementer about Learner Progress

- Elicit the implementer's perspective on learner outcomes.
- Summarize and validate the implementer's perspective.

Next, ask the implementer to assess and describe the progress that the learner has made since the intervention began (or since the last performance feedback session). You may ask this question generally and elicit information on the learner's overall functioning, or you may ask about the learner's progress in relation to the intervention and its specific goal. Asking about the learner's progress provides an opportunity for the implementer to share his or her

---

Quick Tip 10.1. Summarizing and Validating

 Make use of summarizing and validating throughout the performance feedback meeting to facilitate a positive rapport and ensure that the meeting reflects the implementer's perspective. By summarizing and validating, you have the opportunity to clarify and acknowledge the implementer's views. In summarizing, you can pull together the implementer's description and emphasize certain aspects so that the implementer can see how his or her perspective is aligned with the data or discussion. By validating, you are not necessarily agreeing with the implementer's summary, but acknowledging that it is how the implementer feels about the current situation. For example, if the implementer is very frustrated with the learner, you might summarize and validate these statements by highlighting the lack of improvement in learner outcome data. Suggesting that it is understandable that the implementer is disappointed by this limited change and that he or she must really care about the learner's improvement validates the implementer's concerns. Later in the meeting, you could link the implementer's perspective to the need to improve intervention fidelity.

overall impression of the learner's current functioning, prior to a specific review of the data. Later in the performance feedback meeting, you will be able to refer to the implementer's initial impressions when discussing the importance of consistently implementing difficult intervention steps and encouraging the implementer to commit to intervention fidelity (e.g., "You said that you saw the intervention already making a small difference. If we get these additional steps in place, we should really be able to see strong improvements"). During this step, as the implementer shares his or her perspective, summarize and validate these statements. That is, use your own wording to restate what the implementer has said and acknowledge, in a supportive manner, his or her perspective.

Step 4: Review Intervention Fidelity Data

- Review intervention fidelity data.
- Provide positive feedback for consistently implemented steps and note intervention steps that appear to be more challenging to implement.

This step involves reviewing the current intervention fidelity data, verbally and with graphs if possible, to facilitate a shared impression of the current status of intervention fidelity. To do so, provide an initial overall picture of intervention fidelity by describing the data in a neutral and clear fashion. Then highlight the intervention steps that the implementer delivered consistently. Provide praise and positive feedback about the implementer's delivery of these steps. In doing so, you may note the difficulty of delivering particular implementation steps (e.g., "You did a fantastic job providing high rates of praise, which can be challenging to do") or reference the link between implementation and learner behavior (e.g., "I see that you consistently provided reminders at the beginning of a lesson—that's fantastic as it will really orient the learner to the expectations and make him [her] more likely to follow them"). Indicate which intervention steps have been inconsistently implemented and reflect on the implementer's challenges with intervention fidelity. Use an understanding yet firm tone as you list these steps and describe the current levels of implementation (e.g., "It seems like providing tokens frequently has been challenging; it seems to occur once every hour, whereas we'd like tokens to be provided every 15 minutes"). Use the suggestions provided in Quick Tip Box 10.2 (on p. 190) to keep this discussion positive and supportive, even when examining these steps.

Research findings suggest that showing an implementer a graph of his or her intervention fidelity data is a powerful way to communicate the current status of implementation and facilitate improvements (Gilbertson et al., 2007; Sanetti et al., 2007). Based on these results, we suggest sharing a graph of session intervention fidelity if it's possible to do so. This graph should provide a snapshot of how implementation is going overall, and it should efficiently communicate the current status. Further, the graph can be a useful tool on which to track implementation progress and identify days that might be more difficult than others to implement the intervention. In addition, it may be useful to show the implementer a graph of intervention step fidelity. This graph can help quickly identify intervention steps that are comparatively challenging. Chapter 3 describes how to graph these data, and sample graphs, along with the language describing them, are included in the case examples in Chapter 11.

Quick Tip 10.2. Remaining Positive and Supporting When Intervention Fidelity Is Low

 It is easy to feel frustrated when low levels of intervention fidelity continue and the learner is not able to benefit from the intervention. However, it is important to remain positive and supportive of the implementer, while also being firm about the need for improved intervention fidelity. This way, the implementer will be comfortable being open with you about any confusion or difficulty with implementation, and you can be effective when providing positive feedback for steps consistently implemented. Here are some suggestions for remaining positive and supportive when implementation is low:

- *Think small.* Praise the intervention steps that are regularly implemented. Let the implementer know that his or her delivery of these intervention steps demonstrates that he or she may be able to implement other intervention steps consistently as well.
- *Choose wisely.* Focus on improving the implementer's delivery of one or a small set of intervention steps that will have the biggest influence on the learner's outcomes. Once the implementer sees how the intervention can impact learner outcomes, he or she is more likely to agree to add some additional intervention components.
- *Set goals.* Set intermediate implementation goals that will provide an opportunity for the implementer to demonstrate growth and feel successful, while inching toward full implementation. Goal setting is described further in Step 7.
- *Be empathic.* Remember that implementation can be very challenging! Implementers often have a lot of responsibilities to manage and fitting in a new intervention can definitely be difficult. Having this frame of mind will make it easier to be more understanding of implementation difficulties and will allow you to be more effective in problem-solving how to increase implementation.

Step 5: Review Learner Outcome Data and Highlight Progress toward Intervention Goal

- Review learner outcome data by highlighting progress toward the intervention goal.
- Link the learner's progress to intervention fidelity.

To facilitate the discussion and gain a shared impression of the learner's current progress, you will review the current intervention outcome data, verbally and with graphs if possible. To do so, provide an initial overall picture of the learner's current performance by describing these data in a neutral and clear fashion. Review the intervention goal. As mentioned in Chapter 1, an intervention goal is a specific, measurable, and time-relevant benchmark identifying learner progress. Using the intervention goal, it is possible to review ongoing progress and evaluate whether the learner is expected to meet this benchmark. Highlight the importance of this goal for the learner's progress (e.g., "Remember that if he's able to read at this level of fluency, he'll be at grade level and able to keep up with his peers") or as reflective of the implementer's perspective (e.g., "You'll remember that this was a goal that you described as important for her achieve in order for her to engage appropriately in the classroom"). If appropriate, given the data, describe any improvements in the learner's current performance (e.g., "It seems that she was able to stay on-task during science class this week"). State whether the learner is on track or not on track to meet his or her goal.

Link the learner's progress to the intervention fidelity data. To do so, reflect on the relationship between high levels of intervention fidelity and efficient improvements in learner outcomes. For instance, you might say, "These outcome data are not all that surprising; we saw that intervention fidelity has been challenging, so it makes sense that we're not seeing a huge improvement in the learner's performance" or "This modest change in learner outcomes seems aligned with the intervention fidelity data that we reviewed, in that consistent intervention fidelity is so important to improvements in learner performance." Ask the implementer to reflect on the data as well and to share his or her opinion about the learner's response to the intervention so far. Summarize and validate the implementer's perspective and bring the discussion back to the link between intervention fidelity and learner outcomes.

Step 6: Review and Practice Inconsistently Delivered Intervention Steps

- Carefully review those intervention steps that are not delivered consistently.
- Model, practice with the implementer, and provide feedback.

Following the review of intervention fidelity and learner outcome data, turn to the intervention. A clear description of the intervention steps, followed by modeling, practice, and feedback, will ensure that the implementer understands how to correctly deliver these steps. In many cases, lack of understanding or confidence delivering an intervention step is related to low levels of intervention fidelity. To prepare the implementer, describe clearly and specifically how to deliver each of the challenging intervention steps. Referencing an intervention manual or a written intervention plan that highlights the how-to of difficult intervention steps can help enhance your description. After describing each intervention step, confirm that the implementer understands and provide an opportunity for him or her to ask questions.

Next, take the time to model, practice, and provide feedback. Initially, you may be hesitant or uncomfortable engaging in this process with your colleague; however, we highly suggest incorporating it based on research that indicates the potential benefits to intervention fidelity. To make this process feel natural and supportive as you model the intervention, (1) provide examples of how you might deliver particular steps or (2) explain how you might respond to a particular scenario by delivering the intervention (e.g., "If Johnny calls out, I would respond by . . ."). While modeling, describe what you are doing to deliver the intervention with fidelity, linking this description to your review of the intervention steps earlier. Then have the implementer practice; ask him or her what particular steps might look like or how he or she would respond to particular scenarios. Based on the implementer's performance, provide positive and corrective feedback. In doing so, praise the implementer for intervention steps (or aspects of these steps) delivered correctly and provide specific suggestions to improve intervention steps delivered incorrectly. Provide the implementer with sufficient practice so that he or she can comfortably and correctly deliver all of the challenging intervention steps.

Quick Tip 10.3. Reviewing and Practicing Difficult Intervention Steps

 You can decide to review, model, and practice challenging intervention steps individually or together. If the challenging intervention steps are very different, it may be easier to review, model, and practice each step separately. This way, the implementer can clearly learn one intervention step before considering another. If the intervention steps are similar, delivered at the same time, or delivered sequentially, it may be better to review, model, and practice them at the same time so the implementer can capitalize on the similarities or flow and understand how the steps are delivered together.

Step 7: Problem-Solve How to Improve Progress toward the Intervention Fidelity Goal and Obtain the Implementer's Commitment to the Plan

- Review any intervention fidelity challenges and problem-solve as needed.
- Set an intervention fidelity goal to elicit the implementer's commitment.

Once you've established that the implementer understands how to deliver challenging intervention steps (through discussion and practice in the preceding performance feedback step), engage in discussion and problem solving about potential barriers or difficulties the implementer experiences with delivering the intervention with adequate fidelity. Common barriers to intervention fidelity include managing problem behavior, dealing with competing responsibilities, remembering to implement, or fitting intervention steps into the daily routine (Collier-Meek et al., 2016). Summarize and validate the difficulty that the implementer is experiencing and then collaboratively identify feasible strategies to address the particular barriers mentioned. These strategies may involve modifying the intervention steps or materials, scheduling intervention implementation, or developing strategies to support other learners' behavior. Whatever strategies are identified, make sure that the key components of the learner intervention are maintained. If adjustments to the intervention steps are made, make sure to return to Step 6 to practice delivering it with intervention fidelity.

Once intervention fidelity barriers and related strategies have been identified, link the use of the strategies with the implementer's preparation for delivering the intervention. At this time, it may be appropriate to set an explicit intervention fidelity goal (see Quick Tip 10.4 on p. 193 for additional information). Confirm that the implementer is prepared to deliver the challenging intervention steps to increase intervention fidelity levels and support learner outcomes. For instance, you might say, "Based on what we've talked about today, are you feeling ready to deliver this intervention?" Praise the implementer for his or her commitment to intervention fidelity, if he or she indicates readiness. If the implementer indicates a lack of readiness to deliver the intervention, engage in discussion and relevant problem solving to address any concerns. For instance, you may decide to return to implementation planning (Chapter 5) to planfully adjust the intervention to the context, or you

---

Quick Tip 10.4. Setting Intervention Fidelity Goals

 Intervention fidelity goals can provide specific, shared, and manageable benchmarks to facilitate higher levels of intervention fidelity. These goals can be particularly helpful when intervention fidelity is very low, the implementer is overwhelmed, or accountability is needed, because the goals establish clear benchmarks for improvement. Goals may be related to the overall level of intervention fidelity (e.g., average of 85% intervention fidelity next week) or specific intervention steps (e.g., increase level of behavior-specific praise). Use current intervention fidelity data and information about the intervention to set data-driven implementation goals. Make sure the intervention goals are reasonable for the implementer, include the key components of the intervention, and have both an explicit level of intervention fidelity and time range (e.g., next week, by Friday).

---

may choose to model and practice the intervention with the implementer in the implementation context through participant modeling (Chapter 7).

Step 8: Review the Meeting and Thank the Implementer

• Review the meeting discussion and decisions.

• Thank the implementer and close the meeting.

Close the performance feedback session by providing a summary of the meeting. Describe, in particular, the key discussions regarding the current level of intervention fidelity, areas of implementation strength and those in need of improvement, the relationship between intervention fidelity and learner outcomes, how you and the implementer problem-solved ways to improve inconsistently delivered steps, and the intervention fidelity goals to which the implementer agreed. In doing so, you provide a final opportunity to make sure that you and the implementer agree on the key aspects of the meeting and that you are both clear about the next steps to take to facilitate high levels of intervention fidelity. End the meeting positively by thanking the implementer for engaging in the discussion about intervention fidelity and encouraging him or her to be in touch with you if implementation issues arise.

FOLLOW-UP AFTER PERFORMANCE FEEDBACK

To solidify the discussion and the progress made during performance feedback, we suggest that you engage in some activities after the session. Follow-up after performance feedback involves three steps, outlined in Box 10.4 and described in the next paragraph.

Review session notes to ensure that the strategy was delivered as planned. To do so, check the Performance Feedback Guide (Appendix 10.1) and complete a self-assessment using the Fidelity Data Sheet for Performance Feedback (Appendix 10.2) to see if you addressed each of the strategy steps. If you missed any steps, follow up with the implementer. It is important to make sure that the strategies were delivered as planned so that they have the most likelihood of impacting the implementer. If needed, *update the interven-*

> ## BOX 10.4. Follow-Up Steps after Performance Feedback
>
> 1. Review session notes to ensure that the strategy was delivered as planned.
> 2. Update the intervention plan and/or the implementation plan, as needed.
> 3. Check in with the implementer following the meeting to touch base about intervention fidelity and to answer any questions.

tion plan and/or the implementation plan. If any changes were made during performance feedback, update the written materials to reflect those changes. Share the updated materials with the implementer as soon as possible. Last, *check in with implementer following the meeting to touch base about implementation and answer any questions.* This follow-up will ensure that the implementer feels comfortable delivering the intervention after the meeting and that his or her questions have been answered. Confirm that implementer knows how to contact you with any questions about the intervention or its implementation.

ADAPTATIONS TO PERFORMANCE FEEDBACK

For the most part, you will likely deliver performance feedback using all of the steps described above. Even so, the particular context, implementer, and/or intervention may suggest that an adaptation would be useful. When deciding to make adaptations to performance feedback, it is critical that you include the essential steps, while reducing other steps or adding in additional steps. Studies suggest that performance feedback must, at the very least, include Step 4: a review of intervention fidelity data that includes praise for steps consistently implemented and corrective feedback for steps inconsistently delivered (Noell et al., 2014). In our experience, this discussion is more comfortable when it follows a description of the meeting purpose (Step1) and a discussion of the implementer's perspective on intervention implementation (Step 2), and is followed by problem-solving implementation (Step 7) and reviewing the meeting and thanking the implementer (Step 8).

When considering potential adaptations to performance feedback, use Table 10.1 to identify the appropriate combination of components for the context. Whatever combination of components is applied in a performance feedback meeting, make sure to monitor their effectiveness. That is, evaluate any changes to intervention fidelity after engaging in performance feedback with the implementer. It may take a few meetings for the implementer's intervention fidelity to increase, as they may need to time to learn particular intervention steps, come around to intervention fidelity, or understand the implications of the feedback being provided. If improvement has not been observed after a period of time, it may be appropriate to reconsider the performance feedback components being applied or increase the frequency of the meetings.

TABLE 10.1. Adaptations for Performance Feedback

Potential component to performance feedback	What does it involve?	When might it be applied?
Verbal feedback only[a]	• Discuss intervention fidelity, praising strengths and providing corrective feedback for steps delivered inconsistently	• Always; verbal feedback is essential for this implementation support
Graphic feedback[a]	• Show visual, graphic depiction of intervention fidelity across time or by intervention component	• Whenever feasible; most performance feedback evaluated in research includes this component
Learner data review[a]	• Discuss learner progress toward intervention goal and its relationship to intervention fidelity data; may include graphic display	• Whenever feasible; most performance feedback evaluated in research includes this component
Problem solving to support implementation[a]	• Discuss how to address current barriers or issues related to intervention fidelity	• Whenever feasible; most performance feedback evaluated in research includes this component
Goal setting	• Develop a goal for increasing intervention fidelity; may be related to specific intervention steps or overall	• When intervention fidelity is very low, the implementer is overwhelmed, or accountability is needed; use goal setting to identify and monitor manageable targets for improvement
Self-monitoring	• Identify a feasible way for the implementer to monitor his or her intervention fidelity of specific intervention steps or overall	• When the implementer could benefit from ongoing prompts about his or her intervention fidelity and is open to collecting these data
Modeling[a]	• Demonstrate, in person or via video, how to deliver specific intervention steps or the whole intervention; may occur outside or within the target setting	• Whenever feasible; most performance feedback evaluated in research includes this component • Particularly important if intervention fidelity is low because the implementer does not understand how to deliver specific steps

(continued)

TABLE 10.1. *(continued)*

Potential component to performance feedback	What does it involve?	When might it be applied?
Role play	• Demonstrate how to deliver the intervention in response to particular scenarios or situations	• When the implementer understands the intervention steps in isolation, but might benefit from practice of how to implement them together or in difficult situations
Positive reinforcement	• Provide positive acknowledgment or rewards to the implementer contingent on high levels of intervention fidelity	• When the implementer knows how to deliver the intervention, but intervention fidelity remains low and within-meeting praise is not sufficient acknowledgment • When the implementer is motivated by external rewards that can be feasibly obtained
Negative reinforcement	• Allow the implementer to cancel performance feedback meetings or escape another responsibility (e.g., lunch duty), contingent on high levels of intervention fidelity	• When the implementer knows how to deliver the intervention, but intervention fidelity remains low and the implementer is motivated by avoiding the performance feedback sessions or other responsibilities that can be feasibly removed

*a*Step included in typical performance feedback sessions.

SUMMARY

Performance feedback is a form of implementation support that involves meeting with an implementer to review and discuss intervention fidelity data, including what is going well and what is challenging. It may also include a graphic review of intervention fidelity data, discussion of learner outcomes, modeling and practice of intervention steps, and problem solving around intervention fidelity difficulties. Performance feedback has been widely researched and is considered an effective implementation support (Fallon et al., 2015; Noell et al., 2014). Although it can be used across a wide range of implementers, interventions, and situations, performance feedback is particularly recommended for implementers who continue to struggle to deliver an intervention after receiving other, less intensive, implementation supports or when implementers struggle to deliver a high-intensity learner intervention. Use the preceding the step-by-step guide as well as information about potential adaptations and preparation to deliver a supportive and effective performance feedback session.

Performance Feedback Guide

Consultant: _____   Implementer: _____   Date: _____

Learner: _____   Intervention: _____   Start/End Time: _____

READINESS CHECKLIST

✓	**Have you . . .**
	1. Reviewed the intervention and current data?
☐	Familiarized yourself with the intervention plan?
☐	Reviewed the intervention goal and, using data, the learner's current progress?
☐	Evaluated intervention fidelity data?
	2. Prepared to provide performance feedback?
☐	Read about performance feedback?
☐	Practiced dialogue, as needed, to be comfortable at the meeting?
	3. Identified meeting logistics?
☐	Scheduled the performance feedback session?
☐	Reached out to the implementer?
☐	Brought performance feedback materials to the session?

PERFORMANCE FEEDBACK GUIDE

Step 1: Explain the Purpose of the Session

- Provide an overview of performance feedback.
- Begin providing performance feedback in an open, supportive manner.

Following is an example of what you might say to explain the purpose of this session:

> "Today, we're here to discuss how implementing [*intervention*] has been progressing. We're going to talk about what's been working and we'll review and problem-solve any intervention steps or issues that have been challenging."

_____

_____

_____

(continued)

Step 2: Ask the Implementer about Intervention Fidelity

- Elicit the implementer's perspective on intervention fidelity.
- Summarize and validate the implementer's perspective.

  "So, how has intervention implementation been going?" [*Summarize and validate response.*]

_____

_____

_____

Step 3: Ask the Implementer about Learner Progress

- Elicit the implementer's perspective on the learner's outcomes.
- Summarize and validate the implementer's perspective.

  "How is [*learner*] responding to [*intervention*]?" [*Summarize and validate the response.*]

_____

_____

_____

Step 4: Review Intervention Fidelity Data

- Review intervention fidelity data.
- Provide positive feedback for consistently implemented steps and note interventions steps that appear to be more challenging to implement.

  "Let's take a look at the implementation data we've collected. [*Show graph and review implementation strengths.*] You've done an excellent job with [*describe implementation strengths*]. That's fantastic. [*Review implementation inconsistencies.*] I see that [*inconsistently implemented step(s)*] has been challenging to deliver on a regular basis. Is that right?"

_____

_____

_____

(continued)

Step 5: Review Learner Outcome Data and Highlight Progress toward Intervention Goal

- Review the learner outcome data by highlighting progress toward the intervention goal.
- Link the learner's progress to intervention fidelity.

   "Let's take a look at how [*learner*] has been doing. We had a goal for [*learner*] of [*describe learner goal*]. Based on the progress monitoring data [*describe these data*] [*learner*] is [*on track/not on track*] to meet the goal. That's aligned with the implementation data [*link learner progress and intervention fidelity data.*] Does that match what you're seeing?"

_____

_____

_____

Step 6: Review and Practice Inconsistently Delivered Intervention Steps

- Carefully review those intervention steps that are not implemented consistently.
- Model, practice with the implementer, and provide feedback.

   "So, let's take a look at the challenging intervention steps. [*For each intervention step, describe the procedures and when it's to be delivered. Model each step and provide opportunities for practice and feedback as needed.*] Does that make sense?" [*Confirm the implementer's understanding.*]

_____

_____

_____

Step 7: Problem-Solve How to Improve Progress toward the Intervention Fidelity Goal and Obtain the Implementer's Commitment to the Plan

- Review any intervention fidelity challenges and problem-solve as needed.
- Set an intervention fidelity goal to elicit the implementer's commitment.

   "So, based on this information, let's problem-solve how we could improve the implementation of these intervention steps. What challenges can we address? [*Problem-solve.*] Based on what we discussed, it seems that it might be reasonable to [*intervention fidelity goal*]. Does that sound like a plan?" [*Confirm and praise the implementer's commitment to the plan.*]

_____

_____

_____

(continued)

Step 8: Review the Meeting and Thank the Implementer

- Review the meeting discussion and decisions.
- Thank the implementer and close the meeting.

  "We discussed how it's been going with [*intervention*]. You've been doing a great job with [*consistently implemented steps*], and we've reviewed how to deliver [*inconsistently implemented steps*]. We decided on [*implementation goal*] and came up with [*strategies to address challenges*]. Does that sound right? Any other questions? [*Answer any questions.*] Thank you for meeting with me, and remember that you can always reach out with questions or for support."

_____

_____

_____

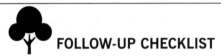 **FOLLOW-UP CHECKLIST**

✓	Have you . . .
☐	1. Reviewed the session notes to ensure that the strategy was delivered as planned?
☐	2. Updated the intervention plan and/or the implementation plan, as needed?
☐	3. Checked in with the implementer following the meeting to touch base about implementation and to answer any questions?

Fidelity Data Sheet for Performance Feedback

For each of the strategy steps, provide a rating of adherence (to what extent you covered each step) and of quality (how well you delivered each step) based on the following rubric.

Adherence	Quality
2 = All components of step delivered. 1 = Some components of step delivered. 0 = No components of step delivered.	2 = Step delivered in a smooth, natural manner, responsive to the implementer, and with appropriate nonverbal interaction. 1 = Step delivered with some aspects of quality. 0 = Step delivered without any aspects of quality.

Strategy Steps	Adherence	Quality
1. Explain the purpose of the session.		
2. Ask the implementer about intervention fidelity.		
3. Ask the implementer about learner progress.		
4. Review intervention fidelity data.		
5. Review learner outcome data and highlight progress toward intervention goal.		
6. Review and practice inconsistently delivered intervention steps.		
7. Problem-solve how to improve progress toward the intervention fidelity goal and obtain the implementer's commitment to the plan.		
8. Review the meeting and thank the implementer.		

First, sum each column: _____ _____

16   16

Next, divide by number of steps to identify a percentage: = _____% = _____%

PART IV

PUTTING IT ALL TOGETHER

CHAPTER 11

Managing Implementation Supports to Improve Student Achievement

with Ashley M. Boyle

Throughout this book we have discussed how to extend the problem-solving model (i.e., identify a learner concern, take baseline data and identify an intervention, implement an intervention, assess learner outcomes) to include intervention implementation assessment and support. Why? Consistent implementation is more likely to result in efficient improvement to learner outcomes, and, the fact is, most implementers need at least some support to be successful. We began with a broad overview of intervention implementation (Chapter 1). Then we provided an overview of the problem-solving model with embedded implementation activities (Chapter 2), and explained how to collect intervention fidelity data (Chapter 3), make subsequent decisions (Chapter 4), and deliver implementation support via a range of performance- and skill-building strategies (Chapters 6–10). We hope that you will use this model as a framework to individualize your intervention fidelity data collection, decisions, and supports appropriate to the learners and implementers in your context.

To illustrate how to put it all together, we provide two case studies. The first case study introduces Kyle, a preschool learner with autism spectrum disorder, and his dedicated education team, including his mother, as they work to provide academic and behavioral support at school and home. The second case study involves three seventh-grade general education students with a range of behavioral and academic concerns, and the team of teachers and other school personnel that is working to support their success through Tier 2 interventions. These case studies highlight the processes of identifying the learner's concern and an appropriate research-based intervention, providing proactive implementation support, collecting intervention fidelity data alongside learner outcome data, and delivering and evaluating targeted implementation support.

Ashley M. Boyle, MA, is doctoral candidate in school psychology at the University of Connecticut and predoctoral intern at Kennedy Krieger in Baltimore, Maryland.

CASE STUDY 1: SUPPORTING STAFF AND PARENTS TO IMPLEMENT A COMPREHENSIVE INTERVENTION PLAN

Phase 1: Prepare

Ms. Smith is a behavior analyst who consults with school staff and families to develop comprehensive intervention programming for young learners with complex needs. She is currently working with Mr. Hall (special education teacher), Ms. Lee and Ms. Garcia (morning and afternoon paraeducators), and Ms. Davis (mother) to develop a behavior support plan (BSP) and functional academic programming for Kyle, a learner with autism spectrum disorder who is newly enrolled in a full-day inclusive preschool program.

Step 1: Identify a Learner Concern

Kyle is an inquisitive learner who has many interests, particularly vehicles and animals. Although his expressive language is limited to words and short phrases at this point, he has a strength in making requests for his wants and needs. Across settings Kyle also demonstrates some interfering problem behaviors. At the initial team meeting with all stakeholders, the team identified target problem behaviors (i.e., disruption with materials, noncompliance, and tantrums) and developed operational definitions (see Figure 11.1). Stakeholders noted that Kyle has the most difficulties during transitions from preferred activities and academic blocks. At home, Ms. Davis notices that these behaviors tend to occur when he has to put away his toys or when she makes demands. Ms. Smith documented the completion of this step on the Implementation Tracking Log (see Figure 11.2).

Stakeholders	

Team:
• Behavior Analyst, Ms. Smith
• Special Education Teacher, Mr. Hall
• Paraeducators:
   o Ms. Lee (morning)
   o Ms. Garcia (afternoon)
• Mother, Ms. Davis
	Learner:
	Kyle, a preschool student with autism spectrum disorder

Learner Concerns	

Learner Concerns
Behavior Concerns: • *Disruption with materials*: Any instance or attempt to swipe, knock over, or throw instructional materials. Each instance or attempt is recorded as a tally. • *Noncompliance*: Any instance in which Kyle fails to comply with demands after two prompts. Each instance or attempt is recorded as a tally. • *Tantrums*: An instance in which Kyle flops to the floor, kicks his legs, and screams and/or cries. An instance is recorded when these behaviors are present for 5 seconds, and it ends in the absence of the behaviors for 15 seconds. A new instance of this behavior can be recorded after the behaviors are absent for 30 seconds.

FIGURE 11.1. Case study 1 overview.

Learner: Kyle

Consultant: Ms. Smith

Implementers: K's school-based team (Mr. Hall, Ms. Lee, Ms. Garcia), mother (Ms. Davis)

Intervention: Behavior support plan and discrete trial instruction

Use this worksheet to document the implementation process.

Date	Activity/Meeting	Action Steps	Person Responsible	Date Due	Notes
Phase 1: Prepare					
9/10	1. Identify a learner concern	• Conduct team meeting to operationalize concerns • Plan to collect baseline data	Consultant Consultant	9/15	
9/15	2. Collect baseline data	• Collect sufficient baseline data • Summarize baseline data	School-based team and consultant Consultant	10/2	
10/2	3. Confirm the concern and set a goal	• Decide if there is a concern to be addressed • Develop SMART goals	Consultant and school-based team Consultant	10/4	
10/4	4. Identify the intervention	• Obtain intervention materials • Develop a draft of intervention fidelity materials	Consultant Consultant	10/11	
10/11	5. Planfully adapt the intervention to the context/resources (i.e., provide implementation planning)	• Share the implementation plan	Consultant	10/14	
10/11	6. Provide high-quality training (i.e., direct training)	• Train the implementers • Make sure the intervention materials are available to the implementers	Consultant Consultant	10/14	

(continued)

FIGURE 11.2. Case study 1 Implementation Tracking Log.

Date	Activity/Meeting	Action Steps	Person Responsible	Date Due	Notes
Phase 2: Implement and Evaluate					
10/14	7. Implement the intervention	• Determine dates for implementation and learner outcome assessment • Add dates for assessment and for data review to the Implementation Tracking Log	Implementers Consultant	11/5	
10/14	8a. Collect learner outcome data	• Graph the data • Interpret the data	Paraeducators Consultant and special education teacher	11/5	
10/14	8b. Collect intervention fidelity data	• Graph and interpret the data • Develop a summary statement	Consultant Consultant	11/5	
11/5	9. Evaluate the intervention and make data-based decisions (use Data-Based Decision-Making Worksheet)	• Identify action steps based on the data profile	Consultant	11/7	
Phase 3: Support (as needed)					
11/7	10. Support implementation	• Provide participant modeling to Ms. Lee • Provide motivational interviewing to Ms. Garcia • Provide completed planning for change worksheet • Enact role playing with Ms. Davis	Consultant and special education teacher Consultant Consultant Consultant	11/16	
11/16	11. Evaluate the intervention	• Evaluate intervention fidelity and learner outcome data	Consultant	11/30	
Repeat Steps 10 and 11 as needed.					
11/30	10. Support implementation	• Provide Ms. Lee with performance feedback	Consultant	12/5	
12/20	11. Evaluate the intervention	• Evaluate intervention fidelity and learner outcome data	Consultant	12/22	

FIGURE 11.2. *(continued)*

Step 2: Collect Baseline Data

The team worked hard to collect meaningful baseline data to inform a functional behavioral assessment (FBA). Ms. Lee and Ms. Garcia, who work one-on-one with Kyle in the morning and afternoon, respectively, recorded the frequency of all target behaviors and the duration of tantrums, as well as information about desired behaviors (e.g., frequency of Kyle's appropriate spontaneous requests for help, breaks, and items; see Figure 11.3). They also indicated what happened before and after each problem behavior. Ms. Davis recorded similar data at home each afternoon from 5 P.M. to 6 P.M., using a clicker for feasibility. During her once weekly consultation, Ms. Smith collected more detailed data on the antecedents, behaviors, and consequences at home and at school, as well as rates of problem ver-

---

Directions: Tally each instance of problem behavior in which Kyle engages. Also record the number of desired behaviors (appropriate requests for help, breaks, and preferred items).

- **Disruption with materials:** Any instance of or attempt to swipe, knock over, or throw instructional or other materials. Any instance of banging on a wall or divider. Each instance or attempt is recorded as a tally.
- **Noncompliance (NC):** Any instance in which Kyle fails to comply with demands after two prompts. Each instance or attempt is recorded as a tally.
- **Tantrums:** An instance in which Kyle flops to the floor, kicks his legs, and screams and/or cries. An instance is recorded when the example behaviors are present for 5 seconds, and it ends in the absence of the behaviors for 15 seconds. A new instance of this behavior can be recorded after the behaviors are absent for 30 seconds.

| Daily Individual Behavior Data |

Time	Activity	Disruption Tally	NC Tally	Tantrums Tally	Req. for Break	Req. for Help	Req. for Item
8:15	Arrival/Breakfast						
8:45	Learning						
10:15	A.M. Recess						
10:30	Learning						
11:30	Lunch						
12:00	Recess						
12:30	Learning						
1:45	Snack/Pack-Up						
Daily Totals							

Tantrum Duration (Minutes and Seconds)							
1		6		11		16	
2		7		12		17	
3		8		13		18	
4		9		14		19	
5		10		15		20	

FIGURE 11.3. Case study 1 baseline data collection form.

sus desired behaviors. Mr. Hall and Ms. Smith conducted curriculum-based and adaptive assessments to learn about Kyle's academic and functional skill areas of strength and where instruction needed to be targeted. Ms. Smith documented the completion of this step on the Implementation Tracking Form (see Figure 11.2).

Step 3: Confirm the Concern and Set a Goal

After data were collected for 2 weeks and consistent patterns were emerging, the team came together to review the summarized data (see Figure 11.4). At school, Kyle engaged in an average of 25 instances of disruption with materials, 30 instances of noncompliance, and 10 tantrums (each lasting an average of 5 minutes) per 7-hour school day. At home, Kyle engaged in an average of 10 instances of disruption with materials, five instances of noncompliance, and two tantrums (each lasting an average of 5 minutes) after school during the 1-hour observation period. Kyle did not request help, breaks, or access to preferred items appropriate across settings. Data from the FBA presented a similar picture for home and at school and are reflected in the following summary statements:

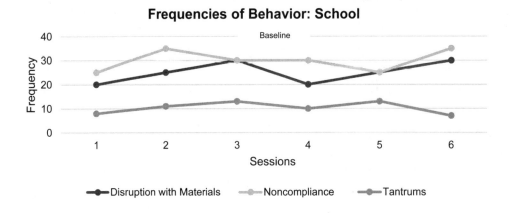

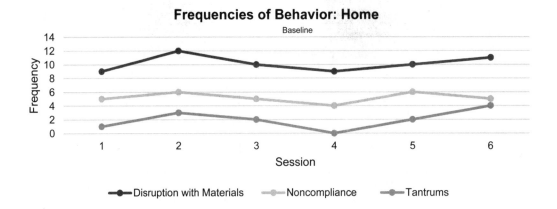

FIGURE 11.4. Learner baseline data at school and home.

- In general, Kyle is more likely to engage in problem behaviors when he is tired or sick.
- When Kyle is presented with nonpreferred, difficult, novel, or high rates of demands, he engages in disruption with materials and through noncompliance to escape the demand.
- When a preferred activity ends or a preferred item is removed, Kyle engages in tantrum behavior to maintain access to the preferred item or activity.

Academic and functional assessments suggested strengths with motor imitation, picture matching, rote counting, tracing, and requesting wants and needs verbally, whereas areas in need of intensive instruction were related to sorting, letter naming and matching, and counting objects. The team collaborated to write SMART (specific, measurable, achievable, relevant, time-bound) goals related to improving Kyle's academic functioning for the target skill areas, reducing levels of problem behavior, and increasing use of replacement behaviors (see Figure 11.5). Ms. Smith documented the completion of this step on the Implementation Tracking Log (see Figure 11.2).

Step 4: Identify an Intervention

Based on the FBA data and further input from the team on Kyle's interests, schedule, and additional skills, as well as their preferences and comfort in implementing different intervention ideas, Ms. Smith developed a functionally relevant BSP to be implemented at school and at home (see Figure 11.6). Additionally, Ms. Smith and Mr. Hall collaborated to develop initial academic programming based on the assessment data and using a discrete trial instruction (DTI) framework with errorless learning procedures, as Kyle did not seem to be responding to less explicit teaching methods (see Figure 11.7). Ms. Smith documented the completion of this step on the Implementation Tracking Log (see Figure 11.2).

Step 5: Planfully Adapt the Intervention to the Context/Resources

SCHOOL

After the behavioral and academic interventions were developed, the team reconvened to review the plan, engage in proactive implementation support, and receive high-quality training. Ms. Smith led the implementation planning session with the school-based team,

> - Given adequate implementation of behavior supports, Kyle will reduce the frequency of the problem behaviors in which he engages by 50% of baseline across settings and maintain this reduction across 80% of days over a 3-week period.
> - Given daily teaching and opportunities to practice, Kyle will increase the number of appropriate replacement behaviors (i.e., requesting breaks, asking for 1 more minute of preferred items/activities) he requests independently to 25% of the total number of replacement behaviors provided (i.e., prompted + independent) across settings and maintain this increase across 80% of days over a 3-week period.

FIGURE 11.5. Case study 1 SMART goals.

Antecedent:
- Display and review daily visual schedule, within-task schedule, and first–then board.
- Provide transition warnings prior to each transition and use a visual timer.
- Provide Kyle with equal choices for the order of academic activities he completes, materials he uses, and reinforcers he earns.
- Prompt behavioral expectations and use of replacement behavior before each new activity, using visual reminders.
- Use preferred and mastered skills, such as gross motor imitation, to create behavioral momentum before difficult tasks.
- Use precise commands to clearly state academic demands and one-step directions.

Teaching and Replacement Behavior:
- Honor Kyle's requests for breaks.
- Honor Kyle's requests for 1 more minute of preferred items/activities (up to three times).
- Teach Kyle how to request and appropriately take breaks using modeling, and practice three times daily when he is not escalated.
- Teach Kyle how to request 1 more minute of preferred items/activities using modeling and practice in the context of reward time.

Reinforcing Replacement and Desired Behavior:
- Use behavior-specific praise each time Kyle engages in a replacement or desired behavior.
- Provide a small reinforcer (e.g., edibles, tickles, 1 minute of access to toys) each time Kyle completes an academic lesson, and a larger reinforcer (e.g., 5 minutes on an iPad, a game, preferred toys) each time Kyle completes a work board (three lessons).
- Provide an edible reinforcer if Kyle appropriately transitions from a preferred activity, or give a preferred item/toy to an adult at the end of reward time.

Responding to Problem Behavior:
- Ignore or neutrally/nonverbally redirect problem behaviors using a visual display of behavioral expectations.
- Ensure that Kyle completes the task before he accesses preferred items/activities.
- If Kyle engages in high rates of problem behavior (i.e., three or more disruptions with materials during one academic lesson, any unsafe behaviors), prompt him to take a 1-minute break in a designated space. Do not provide attention or access to materials during this time and immediately re-present his work after the break is over.

FIGURE 11.6. Case study 1 behavior support plan summary.

- Gather the needed materials.
- Gain the student's attention prior to presenting the demand.
- Use precise commands.
- Implement least-to-most prompting procedure.
- Provide behavior-specific praise for each correct response.
- Provide tokens on token board for each correct response.
- Provide specific error corrections.
- Provide rewards after token board is complete.
- Teach to the correct target.
- Follow the lesson script.
- Collect data on academic responses (i.e., correct, prompted, incorrect).

FIGURE 11.7. Case study 1 discrete trial instruction summary.

during which the team planfully adapted intervention components to the specific context, embedded implementer preferences, documented these modifications, engaged in logistical planning (including who was responsible for obtaining and developing resources), identified possible barriers to successfully implementing the BSP and DTI sessions, and brainstormed strategies to address these barriers. In regard to BSP modifications, the team preferred the replacement behavior of asking for a break over asking to be finished, so this change was reflected in the updated plan. A sampling of the Action Plan Worksheet (prevention strategies) as well as the full Coping Planning Worksheet is provided in Figure 11.8 (see Appendix 5.2). Following the meeting, a copy of the Summary Report for Implementation Planning (Appendix 5.4) was provided to all team members. Ms. Smith completed the corresponding Fidelity Data Sheet for Implementation Planning (Appendix 5.3) to document that the team received the implementation plan as written and documented the provision of the support on the Implementation Tracking Log (see Figure 11.2).

HOME

Ms. Smith met with Ms. Davis in the home setting to review the modifications to the school BSP for the home setting and conduct implementation planning with her. Through this support, Ms. Davis better understood how to integrate delivering the plan with the typical evening routine. Ms. Smith completed the corresponding Fidelity Data Sheet for Implementation Planning (Appendix 5.3) to document that Ms. Davis received the implementation planning as written and documented the provision of this support in the Implementation Tracking Log (see Figure 11.2). She sent a copy of the implementation plan to Ms. Davis shortly after they met.

Step 6: Provide High-Quality Training

SCHOOL

After implementation planning was completed, Ms. Smith provided direct training on all elements of the BSP (i.e., prevention, teaching strategies, replacement behaviors, reinforcement, and responsive strategies), and utilized ample opportunities for modeling, practice, and feedback for each school-based implementer (e.g., Mr. Hall, Ms. Lee, and Ms. Garcia). Mr. Smith and Ms. Hall similarly led the paraeducators through direct training for each DTI lesson, focusing on the prompting and error-correction procedures. Ms. Smith completed the corresponding Fidelity Data Sheet for Direct Training (Appendix 6.2) to document that the team received direct training as planned and documented the provision of this support on the Implementation Tracking Log (see Figure 11.2).

HOME

Ms. Smith also provided direct training to Ms. Davis. During this strategy, Ms. Davis learned and practiced how to deliver the plan with fidelity. At the end of the session, Ms. Smith completed the corresponding Fidelity Data Sheet for Direct Training (Appendix 6.2)

Action Plan					
Intervention Step	**To Be Implemented**				**Resources Needed?**
	When?	**How Often?**	**For How Long?**	**Where?**	
Use daily visual schedule	Review at the beginning of the day, and reference throughout the day	Put up entire schedule at beginning of the day; take down activities after they've occurred	< 5 minutes to review at the beginning of the day, < 1 minute after each activity	Learner workspace	Construction paper, picture icons for all activities (to be laminated)
Use within-task schedule	During all academic times	Make new board after the completion of three lessons and corresponding reward time	< 2 minutes to make a new board and review	At desk	Construction paper (to be laminated)
Use first–then board	Throughout the day	Modify after the completion of each activity	< 1 minute to change and review	Throughout the building	Icons for work, reward options, recess, lunch, specials (to be laminated)
Provide transition warnings	Before the end of each preferred activity	One minute before the end of the activity	< 1 minute	Throughout the building	Visual timer
Provide equal choices	Throughout the day	Every opportunity (order of activities, materials to use, reward options, etc.)	< 1 minute each time	Throughout the building	N/A
Prompt behavioral expectations	Throughout the day, particularly before academics and at end of reward time	Throughout the day	< 1 minute each time	Throughout the building	Visual of behavioral expectations (to be laminated)
Use behavioral momentum	Before particularly difficult tasks	Before each difficult academic sequence of tasks	< 2 minutes each time	Learner workspace, reward area	N/A
Prompt replacement behavior	Academics and reward time	Before each difficult sequence of tasks (break), before each transition from preferred activity (1 more minute)	< 1 minute each time	Throughout the building	Visual of replacement behaviors (e.g., break card, 1 more minute icon; to be laminated)
Use precise commands	Throughout the day	Every time you make an academic or nonacademic request	< 1 minute each time	Throughout the building	N/A

Coping Plan	
Potential Major Barrier to Intervention Implementation	**Strategy to Implement the Intervention Nevertheless**
It could be difficult to remember to implement all the steps	Embed visual prompts throughout the classroom as reminders to implement intervention steps (e.g., a list of key intervention steps in Kyle's workspace and other key locations)
Not enough time in the day to fit in all activities (behavior supports, academic lessons, and inclusion activities)	Make explicit schedule for when certain activities need to occur and options for other times; review for feasibility after 1 week
Other learners might get jealous of all the things Kyle is earning and act out	Explain that every learner needs something different to help him or her do his or her best in school; consider a classwide reinforcement system so all are earning points for appropriate behavior
Data collection can be challenging	Retrain on data collection methods; buy clickers for frequency counts to be transferred to a data sheet when convenient

FIGURE 11.8. Case study 1 action and coping plans.

to document that Ms. Davis received this support as planned and documented the provision of this support on the Implementation Tracking Log (see Figure 11.2).

Phase 2: Implement and Evaluate

Step 7: Implement the Intervention

After the proactive implementation supports were provided, intervention products were finalized, and materials were gathered, the team initiated implementation at school and home. Ms. Smith documented this step on the Implementation Tracking Log (see Figure 11.2).

Step 8a: Assess Learner Outcomes

Ms. Lee and Ms. Garcia continued to record daily behavior data across the school day, and Ms. Davis collected data after school at home, using the same format as during the baseline data collection period. Data were also collected daily on the use of replacement behaviors (e.g., independent requests for breaks). Ms. Lee and Ms. Garcia conducted DTI sessions with Kyle at specified times of the day, using the lesson plans that Ms. Smith and Mr. Hall developed. The paraeducators also collected data on the correct responses made by Kyle during each lesson and summarized their data as a percentage of trials correct. All behavior and academic data were entered into a spreadsheet on a twice-weekly basis by the paraeducators to generate updated graphs to be visually analyzed by Ms. Smith and Mr. Hall. Ms. Smith documented this step on the Implementation Tracking Log (see Figure 11.2).

Step 8b: Assess Intervention Fidelity

In addition to learner outcome data, intervention fidelity data were collected using multiple methods and sources. To develop the intervention fidelity assessment forms, Ms. Smith listed all essential components of the intervention steps (separated for BSP and DTI), chose the assessment method (direct observation and self-report), and identified rating options. Multiple methods of assessment, including direct assessment, were chosen to collect intervention fidelity data, as this was a fairly intensive intervention that needed to be implemented consistently to achieve desired outcomes (see Figure 11.9). Lack of student response or worsening outcomes might lead to a change in learner placement, so data needed to be collected and reviewed regularly. Direct observations would help Ms. Smith identify possible areas on which to focus if further implementation support was needed. However, this is a resource-intensive assessment method, so self-report was used to supplement the information and provide a space for implementers to ask questions.

　　Likert scales for implementation of BSP and DTI components were developed for direct observation ratings, with operational definitions provided for what adherence ("Implemented as planned, "Implemented with deviation," "Not implemented") and quality ("Good," "Fair," "Poor") looked like for each intervention step; a summary score was calculated for the percentage of steps rated "Implemented as planned" (see Figure 11.10). At

Direct Observation	Self-Report
• Collect Likert scale data on adherence and quality of each BSP and DTI step. • Ms. Smith collects twice-weekly; 30-minute observations on BSP fidelity for each school-based implementer. • Ms. Smith observes implementation at home three times a week for 30 minutes each time. • Mr. Hall observes each paraeducator implement DTI three times a week.	• Complete the checklist (Yes, Sometimes, No) to measure adherence of each BSP and DTI step. • Completed by each implementer daily at a consistent time.

FIGURE 11.9. Case study 1 intervention fidelity data collection plan.

Date	Time		Activity		Implementer			
Intervention Step	**Adherence**			Not Observed	**Quality**			
	Implemented as Planned	Implemented with Deviation	Not Implemented		Good	Fair	Poor	
1. Gather materials	3	2	1	NA	3	2	1	
2. Gain student attention	3	2	1	NA	3	2	1	
3. Use precise commands	3	2	1	NA	3	2	1	
4. Implement least-to-most prompting	3	2	1	NA	3	2	1	
5. Provide behavior-specific praise	3	2	1	NA	3	2	1	
6. Provide tokens	3	2	1	NA	3	2	1	
7. Provide specific error corrections	3	2	1	NA	3	2	1	
8. Provide rewards after token board is complete	3	2	1	NA	3	2	1	
9. Teach to correct target	3	2	1	NA	3	2	1	
10. Follow lesson script	3	2	1	NA	3	2	1	
11. Collect data on academic responses	3	2	1	NA	3	2	1	
% Implemented as Planned:			**% "Good" Quality:**					

FIGURE 11.10. DTI direct observation form.

the beginning of implementation, Ms. Smith planned to conduct twice-weekly 30-minute observations on BSP fidelity for each school-based implementer, and Mr. Hall observed each paraeducator implement lessons from the DTI programming twice weekly. Both Mr. Hall and Ms. Smith had a consistent observation schedule (i.e., collecting data on the same days and times each week), which aligned with times when staff recorded self-report data. The observation schedule was intended to be faded once implementers demonstrated sufficient and consistent fidelity and accuracy in their self-reporting. Mr. Hall also reviewed the number of lessons that the paraeducators completed with Kyle as a measure of exposure to DTI. Ms. Smith worked with Ms. Davis after school three times a week, conducting direct observations for 30 minutes during each visit, to support Kyle's behavior at home.

Self-report data were collected across implementers (see Figure 11.11). The same list of BSP and DTI steps that were on the direct observation measures were listed to create a simpler checklist format (Yes, Sometimes, No) to measure adherence. These were completed daily, immediately after a 30-minute period in the morning and afternoon, when Kyle's inter-

Each day at the end of the predetermined rating period, reflect on how well you implemented Kyle's behavior support plan strategies. These data will be used to better support you and Kyle.	
Preventive Strategies	
Did I consistently use a daily visual schedule, within-task schedule, and first–then board?	Yes / Sometimes / No
Did I consistently provide transition warnings and use a visual timer?	Yes / Sometimes / No
Did I provide equal choices in the schedule and with reinforcers?	Yes / Sometimes / No
Did I prompt behavioral expectations with visuals before each change in activity?	Yes / Sometimes / No
Did I use behavioral momentum procedures?	Yes / Sometimes / No
Did I state requests and use precise commands?	Yes / Sometimes / No
Replacement Behaviors	
Did I provide at least three opportunities for Kyle to practice taking breaks each day?	Yes / Sometimes / No
Did I regularly prompt Kyle to ask for a break during instructional activities?	Yes / Sometimes / No
Did I regularly prompt Kyle to ask for 1 more minute during preferred activities?	Yes / Sometimes / No
Did I honor all requests for replacement behaviors?	Yes / Sometimes / No
Response Strategies: Praise, Reinforcemnt, and Consequences	
Did I provide high rates of behavior-specific praise?	Yes / Sometimes / No
Did I provide small, tangible reinforcement for appropriate transitions and for discontinuing use of highly preferred items when asked?	Yes / Sometimes / No
Did I provide rewards for completing nonacademic demands based on the written protocol?	Yes / Sometimes / No
Did I provide rewards for completing academic activities based on the written protocol?	Yes / Sometimes / No
Did I use less intensive consequence strategies (planned ignoring, nonverbal cuing) before more intensive (error corrections, staff initiated breaks)?	Yes / Sometimes / No
Did I follow procedures and criteria to prompt a break?	Yes / Sometimes / No
Did I provide specific, brief, and calm constructive feedback/reprimands?	Yes / Sometimes / No

FIGURE 11.11. BSP self-report implementation checklist.

fering problem behavior was most likely to occur and when the DTI sessions were scheduled to be implemented. These also corresponded to times when direct observations were conducted by Ms. Smith and Mr. Hall. Setting up the self-report schedule so that ratings were recorded immediately after a set time of implementation is important in increasing the likelihood of accurate reporting. Aligning the self-report schedule with when Ms. Smith observed would also provide an opportunity for her to give feedback on the accuracy of implementers' self-reporting. The self-report was also completed during a challenging time behaviorally for Kyle, when strategies should be implemented more frequently and implementation might be more difficult in general. Ms. Davis also completed a daily self-report. The self-report was framed as a reflection tool to aid in further developing the contextual fit of the intervention; it provided a chance for implementers to write down anything they wanted clarified about the plans, to better guide implementation support sessions. Ms. Smith and Mr. Hall trained each implementer on how to accurately complete the self-report forms, using modeling and practice of scoring based on vignettes and demonstrations of implementation. Ms. Smith documented this step on the Implementation Tracking Log (see Figure 11.2).

Step 9: Evaluate the Intervention and Make a Data-Based Decision

Learner outcome and intervention fidelity data were entered into a database at the end of each week and were subsequently graphed and visually analyzed by Ms. Smith. After 3 weeks of implementation, Ms. Smith saw little improvement in Kyle's behavioral or academic outcomes at school or at home (see Figure 11.12). To determine if implementation was adequate, Ms. Smith summarized intervention fidelity data (direct observation of adherence and quality) in terms of overall implementation level (session fidelity) and by individual intervention components (intervention step fidelity). She reviewed the level, variability, and trend of the data and decided whether the intervention was delivered to the extent where it could be reasonably expected to benefit the learner. In evaluating both learner outcome and intervention fidelity data together, Data Profile C appeared: Kyle was improving slightly (about a 5% reduction in problem behaviors), but not enough to be on track to meet his goals (i.e., 50% reduction in problem behaviors), and the intervention fidelity across most implementers was insufficient. More specifically, the data revealed the following information.

MS. LEE, KYLE'S MORNING PARAEDUCATOR (SEE FIGURE 11.13)

- Ms. Lee implemented the BSP with a low to moderate level of adherence (average: 50%, range: 40–55%) and variable quality (range: 50–75%).

- Ms. Lee similarly implemented DTI with a low level of adherence (average: 40%, range: 30–60%) and a moderate level of quality (average: 60%, range: 50–70%).

- Based on these data, Ms. Lee showed a skill deficit in implementing the BSP and DTI sessions, as there were some steps of the plans that she was not implementing (e.g., prevention steps, redirecting using visuals, providing rewards for completing academic activities, giving tokens during DTI sessions on a set schedule, following errorless learning procedures) and some steps that she implemented with low levels of quality.

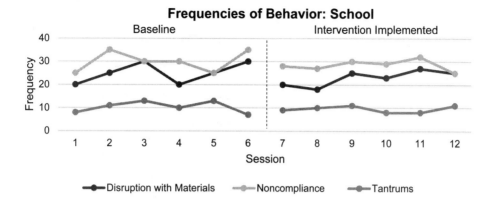

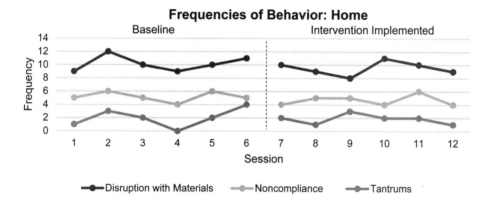

FIGURE 11.12. Learner outcome data after intervention implementation at school and home.

- She was providing Kyle with the target number of DTI sessions across lesson type, which were written in Kyle's schedule, so exposure to DIT lessons was not a concern.

MS. GARCIA, KYLE'S AFTERNOON PARAEDUCATOR (SEE FIGURE 11.14)

- Ms. Garcia implemented the BSP with variable adherence (range: 50–100%) and high levels of quality, which were on an increasing trend (average: 90%, range: 80–100%).

- Ms. Garcia implemented DTI with high levels of adherence (average: 90%, range: 85–100%) and a high level of quality (average: 95%, range: 90–100%).

- Based on these data, Ms. Garcia demonstrated a performance deficit with BSP implementation. During some observations she demonstrated adequate implementation across intervention components, but was inconsistent across observations. She implemented with high levels of quality. She also had more experience implementing DTI, and Mr. Hall's academic fidelity data showed her implementing with adequate fidelity across these sessions.

- She was also providing Kyle with the indicated number of DTI sessions across lesson type.

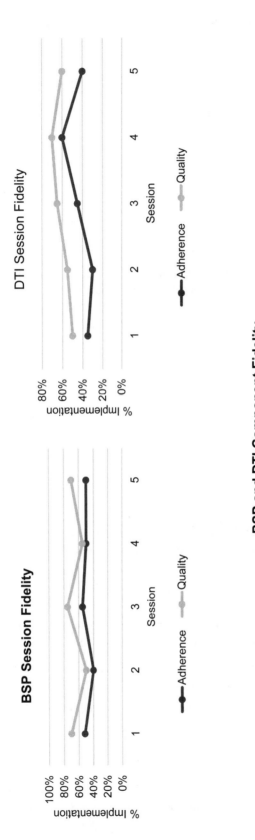

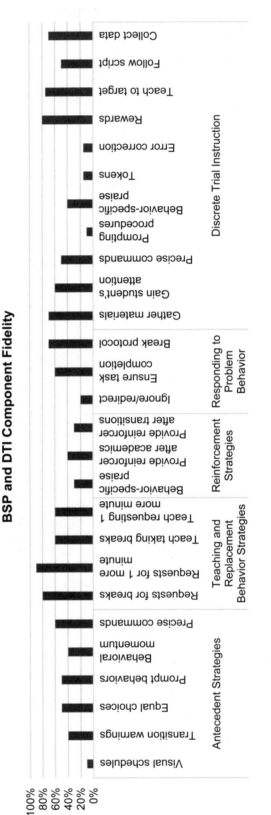

FIGURE 11.13. Ms. Lee's intervention fidelity data after direct training and implementation planning.

220

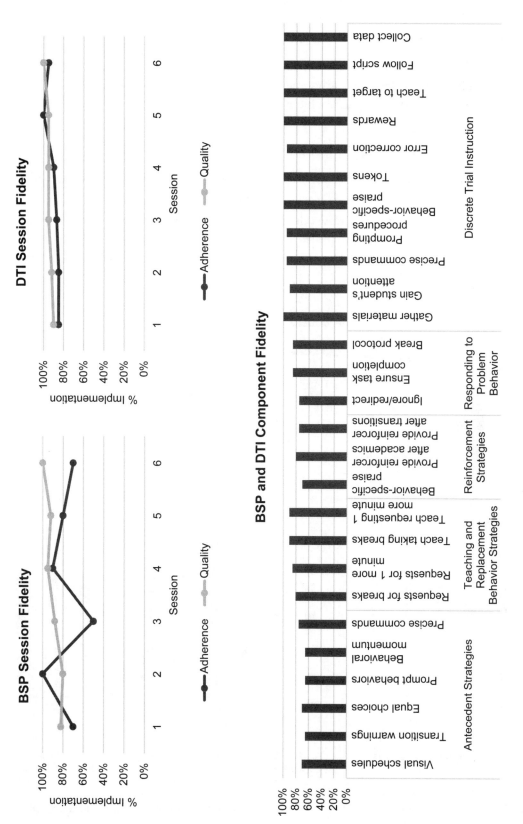

FIGURE 11.14. Ms. Garcia's intervention fidelity data after direct training and implementation planning.

MR. HALL, SPECIAL EDUCATION TEACHER (SEE FIGURE 11.15)

- Mr. Hall was implementing Kyle's BSP with consistent and adequate levels of intervention fidelity, both in terms of adherence (average: 90%, range: 85–100%) and quality (average: 95%, range: 90–100%) across intervention steps.

MS. DAVIS, KYLE'S MOTHER (SEE FIGURE 11.16)

- Ms. Davis implemented the BSP with moderate levels of adherence (average: 65%, range: 50–70%) and a moderate level of quality (average: 70%, range: 60–75%).

- Based on these data, Ms. Davis demonstrated a skill deficit with some BSP steps, such as providing behavior-specific praise, using precision commands, and providing access to replacement behaviors. These steps were not being implemented consistently or with high levels of quality.

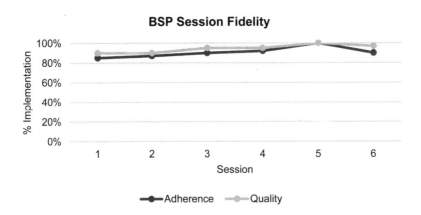

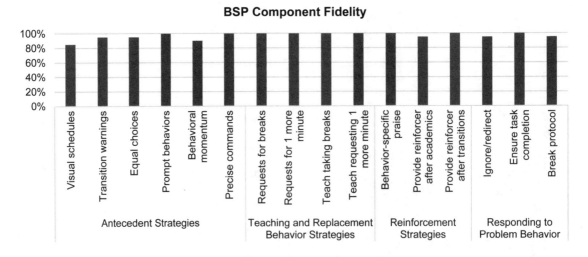

FIGURE 11.15. Mr. Hall's intervention fidelity data after direct training and implementation planning.

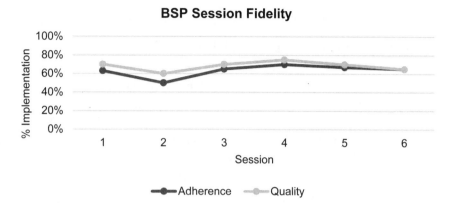

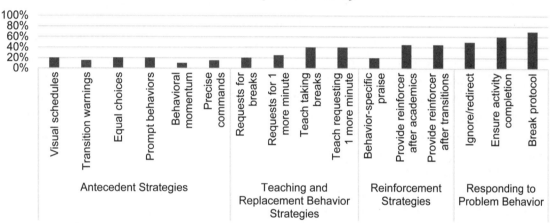

FIGURE 11.16. Ms. Davis's intervention fidelity data after direct training and implementation planning.

Based on these data, targeted implementation supports were identified and provided. Ms. Smith documented next steps in the Data Profile Action Steps Worksheets (Appendix 4.1) and continued to use this form as she provided implementation support. She also documented this step on the Implementation Tracking Form (see Figure 11.2).

Phase 3: Support

Step 10: Implementation Support

Based on the intervention fidelity data, Ms. Lee, Ms. Garcia, and Ms. Davis required additional implementation support.

MS. LEE: SKILL-BUILDING IMPLEMENTATION SUPPORT—PARTICIPANT MODELING

Ms. Lee required supports to address her skill deficit with implementing the BSP and DTI sessions. Ms. Smith and Mr. Hall decided that providing participant modeling for the BSP and DTI lessons would be an appropriate and effective implementation support for Ms. Lee to address her skill deficit, as it provided more opportunities for modeling and practice to promote correct and fluent implementation of intervention steps. Further, the *in vivo* element would be feasible, and it was hypothesized that it would be most helpful for Ms. Lee to see the strategies fully implemented in context with Kyle. Before meeting, Ms. Smith and Mr. Hall set up three sessions with Ms. Lee (the first and third outside of the implementation setting and the second happening *in vivo*), reviewed the intervention rationale, reviewed the intervention fidelity and outcome data, determined intervention steps to target, decided on a tentative order for modeling the intervention steps, and gathered materials. During the *in vivo* portion, Ms. Smith would provide support on BSP components and Mr. Hall would focus on promoting DTI steps, as he had expertise in this area.

Ms. Smith and Mr. Hall met with Ms. Lee to explain the purpose of participant modeling (Step 1) and discuss the intervention and the importance of consistent implementation on learner outcomes (Step 2). They focused their efforts on reviewing the intervention steps that Ms. Lee had demonstrated the most difficulty in implementing (i.e., prevention steps, redirecting using visuals, providing rewards for completing academic activities, giving tokens during DTI sessions on a set schedule, following errorless learning procedures) (Step 3). These steps were prioritized for demonstration during the *in vivo* session, and the team agreed that demonstrating all applicable intervention steps would be most natural and helpful in promoting Ms. Lee's implementation adherence and quality (Step 4). They planned for the *in vivo* exercise to take place the following day during the 9–10 A.M. learning block, during which both the BSP and DTI procedures would be implemented with Kyle (Step 5). During the *in vivo* session, Ms. Smith implemented the BSP components, while Mr. Hall demonstrated correct implementation of DTI (Step 6). This took place for about 20 minutes. The group then transitioned to supported practice, during which Ms. Lee implemented the interventions, while Ms. Smith and Mr. Hall observed and provided prompts to indicate where some intervention steps could be implemented, with feedback (Step 7). After 20 minutes, Ms. Lee implemented the plan with Kyle independently (Step 8). Ms. Smith and Mr. Hall provided feedback on Ms. Lee's implementation and suggested increasing the frequency with which she provided choices and prompted behavioral expectations (Step 9). Ms. Smith then observed Ms. Lee successfully implement the suggestions during a transition and reward time. During the feedback session, Ms. Lee stated that she felt much more confident in implementing the intervention, particularly with giving precise commands and error corrections, and that it was helpful to see it modeled with Kyle (Step 10). Ms. Smith and Mr. Hall noted that they saw a great improvement with the implementation of DTI, particularly with providing specific praise, giving precise commands, recording accurate data, and providing error corrections. Ms. Lee asked many questions regarding implementation in different scenarios; Ms. Smith and Mr. Hall thanked Ms. Lee for letting them model during learning time and for her willingness to try participant modeling (Step 11). Ms. Smith completed the corresponding Fidelity Data Sheet for Participant Modeling

(Appendix 7.3) to document that Ms. Lee received participant modeling as planned, and she documented the provision of this support on the Implementation Tracking Log (see Figure 11.2).

MS. GARCIA: PERFORMANCE-BUILDING IMPLEMENTATION SUPPORT— MOTIVATIONAL INTERVIEWING

Ms. Garcia's implementation difficulties were related to a performance deficit with implementing the BSP. To address this, Ms. Smith chose to use motivational interviewing with Ms. Garcia. Before meeting with Ms. Garcia, Ms. Smith reviewed the implementation data, made a list of benefits for delivering the intervention, and made a "cheat sheet" of open-ended questions to guide the session. Ms. Smith scheduled a time to meet with Ms. Garcia to discuss the delivery of the BSP and to elicit her perspectives on how things were going. To facilitate this discussion, Ms. Garcia said it might be helpful to bring the implementation plan and her self-report forms. During the meeting, Ms. Smith first explained that they were going to talk about how implementing the BSP for Kyle was going (Step 1). Ms. Smith used open-ended questions to find out Ms. Garcia's perceptions of the intervention implementation (i.e., "What's going the best for you in this intervention?"; "What parts is Kyle reacting to the most positively?"; "Are there any parts you would like to be better at delivering?") (Step 2), and summarized these perceptions, while validating change talk (Step 3). For example, Ms. Garcia summarized her perceptions: She noticed that Kyle transitions from preferred activities better when he is prompted to request 1 more minute, and she thinks he responds well to praise and visuals, but she sometimes finds it difficult to remember to implement all the prevention strategies. In turn, Ms. Smith responded: "It seems like implementation of the 1-more-minute protocol, praise, and visuals really help Kyle be successful. You also find it challenging to remember to deliver some of the prevention strategies. Does that sound right?" Ms. Smith reviewed the implementation plan with Ms. Garcia and showed her graphs of her observation fidelity data (Step 4). Ms. Smith asked Ms. Garcia what she noticed when she looked at the data, to which Ms. Garcia responded, "Hmmm . . . it looks like I'm not doing the same thing every day; some days I'm using all of the intervention strategies, but others not so much." Ms. Smith continued to ask Ms. Garcia open-ended questions about the data (e.g., "What is different on days that are better?"; "How might things be different if you implemented the entire BSP each day?"; "How were things different when you did implement the BSP as planned?") and summarized her responses. Ms. Smith then asked Ms. Garcia, "On a scale from 0 to 10, with '0' being 'not at all important' and '10' being 'extremely important,' how important do you think it is for you to deliver Kyle's BSP as we planned?" (Step 5). Ms. Garcia responded with '7,' and Ms. Smith summarized this rating ("A 7—it seems like implementing this intervention is pretty important to you"; Step 6). When questioned why her rating wasn't a '5,' Ms. Garcia responded, "Well, sometimes Kyle does OK even when all the pieces aren't implemented, but then other times I've seen him do really well when I use all the strategies." Ms. Smith asked Ms. Garcia about her perspective on the benefits of implementing the intervention (Step 7). Ms. Smith then shared the list of benefits, developed prior to the meeting, to implementing the BSP with high intervention fidelity, focusing on the benefits that both she and Ms. Garcia came up with (i.e., a decrease in problem behavior, an increase in academic skills, knowing how to appropriately ask for breaks now, finding it easier to engage in appropriate behavior, and learning new skills; Step 8). When Ms. Garcia was asked which benefit to implementing the BSP was the most important and relevant to her, she said that having more time to focus on providing Kyle's academic skill instruction and spending less time on managing behavior were most important to her (Step 9). Ms. Garcia then rated her confidence in her ability to deliver the intervention as an 8 (Step 10). After Ms. Smith summarized and asked why it wasn't a lower number, Ms. Garcia said that she had implemented similar plans in the past and is comfortable with the strategies, but is more unsure of how to handle things when Kyle is having a really tough morning working with Ms. Lee and that behavior carries over into the afternoon. Ms. Smith summarized Ms. Garcia's change talk (e.g., how she views implementing the intervention as important, the many benefits she listed about implementing the intervention, that sometimes it's difficult to implement the intervention after Kyle has had a difficult morning; Step 11) and asked her, "What do you think a good next step would be?" (Step 12). Ms. Garcia indicated that she probably needed to focus on implementing the entire intervention every day, throughout the time she works with Kyle in the afternoon, so he can continue to make progress. They continued with the motivational interviewing session by completing the planning-for-change worksheet (Step 13; see Figure 11.17). Ms. Smith concluded the meeting by reviewing the discussion and decisions (Step 14). She also completed the corresponding Fidelity Data Sheet for Motivational Interviewing (Appendix 9.3) to certify that Ms. Garcia received motivational interviewing as planned, documented the provision of this support on the Implementation Tracking Log (see Figure

The changes I want to make (or continue making) are:
Work on providing the preventive strategies (prompting expectations, reviewing schedule, providing choices, using behavioral momentum) more frequently, especially when Kyle has a difficult morning.
The reasons why I want to make these changes are:
To continue to promote learner success, both behaviorally and academically.
The steps I plan to take in changing are:
Provide honest ratings on my self-report data sheet and reflect on what went well and what didn't for the day, check in with Ms. Lee before we transition to see how Kyle's morning went and plan accordingly (increase use of strategies if he had a difficult time), possibly tally the times that strategies aren't being as consistently implemented.
The ways other people can help me are:
Add section on self-report sheet where I can write what went well and what was difficult to implement each day, as well as a section for questions to be reviewed at weekly team meetings.
I will know if my plan is working if:
I have less variable and higher levels of implementation data. Look at graphs and aim for at least 80% implementation each day—this will lead to improvements in Kyle's behavior.
Some things that could interfere with my plan are:
New or increase in problem behavior—I would be unsure of how to address.
What I will do if the plan isn't working:
Review implementation plan and ask for more support.

FIGURE 11.17. Ms. Garcia's planning-for-change worksheet.

11.2), and checked in with Ms. Garcia a couple of days later to answer any questions and see how her plan was going.

MS. DAVIS: SKILL-BUILDING IMPLEMENTATION SUPPORT—ROLE PLAY

Ms. Davis demonstrated skill deficits in implementing the BSP at home, showing particular difficulty with giving high rates of behavior-specific praise, using precise commands, and providing access to replacement behaviors. Given the skill deficits, Ms. Smith decided to support Ms. Davis using role play. Ms. Davis had described several contexts in which Kyle's behavior was difficult to manage, and role play would provide an opportunity to practice implementation under varying hypothetical circumstances. Before meeting with Ms. Davis, Ms. Smith reviewed the intervention rationale and the intervention fidelity and outcome data, determined intervention steps to be targeted, decided on a tentative order for role-playing target intervention steps, and gathered materials. During the role play meeting, Ms. Smith first explained the purpose of this implementation support (Step 1). Ms. Smith and Ms. Davis then discussed the intervention components and the importance of consistent implementation to improve Kyle's behavior (Step 2). They reviewed the home outcome data and the intervention fidelity data, focusing on the steps that were the most challenging for Ms. Davis to implement consistently (i.e., providing behavior-specific praise, precise commands, and replacement behaviors; Step 3). They chose these, along with redirecting behavior using visual aids and behavioral momentum, as intervention steps to practice (Step 4). Ms. Davis explained that she has the most difficulty implementing the steps during Kyle's bedtime routine, when running errands, and when Kyle has playdates with his cousins (Step 5). She provided further detail on the specific scenarios, and Ms. Smith demonstrated the intervention steps, with Ms. Davis imitating Kyle's typical behavior (Step 6). They brainstormed a few modifications for the different scenarios, which they documented in the implementation plan (Step 7). For her practice, Ms. Davis wanted to make sure that she used high rates of behavior-specific praise, used the proper procedures to provide a break, and practiced these strategies in the context of going to the grocery store. They decided to use the kitchen environment for Ms. Davis to practice her skills. Ms. Smith imitated the kinds of behavior Kyle would display under the circumstances and provided Ms. Davis with some prompts about when to use more proactive strategies (Step 8). After the practice, Ms. Smith noted that Ms. Davis had provided high rates of specific praise and used appropriate procedures to prompt and provide the replacement behaviors (Step 9). Ms. Davis said that she felt more confident implementing these strategies now, and Ms. Smith thanked her for participating in the implementation support (Step 10). Ms. Smith then completed the corresponding Fidelity Data Sheet for Role Play (Appendix 7.4) to note that Ms. Davis had engaged in role play as planned, and that she (Ms. Smith) also documented the provision of this support on the Implementation Tracking Log (see Figure 11.2).

Step 11: Evaluate the Intervention

Two weeks after implementation supports were provided, Ms. Smith reviewed the learner outcome (see Figure 11.18) and intervention fidelity data. Kyle's behavioral incidents in the

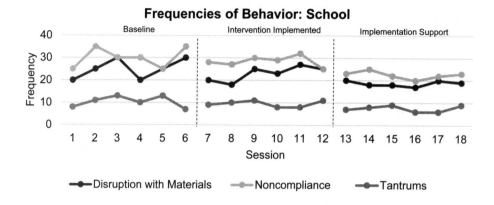

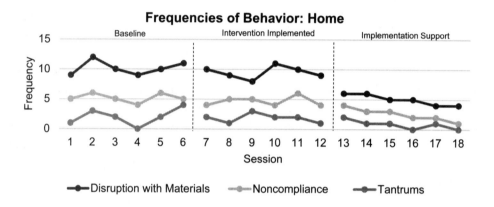

FIGURE 11.18. Learner outcomes after implementation support at school and home.

home environment had decreased substantially, and he was on track to meet his goal in that setting. Ms. Davis's implementation data had also improved to consistent high levels for adherence and quality following the provision of role play (see Figure 11.19). This pattern reflects Data Profile A, and so, following the appropriate action steps, implementation and data collection continued.

Similarly, Ms. Garcia had shown great strides in the consistency with which she implemented the BSP, and Kyle's outcome data reflected the improved implementation in the afternoon (see Figure 11.20 on p. 230). Again, Data Profile A was indicated, and so, following the appropriate action steps, implementation and data collection continued.

Although Ms. Lee's intervention fidelity had improved in providing DTI, she still was not consistently implementing the BSP with high levels of fidelity, and recent data were trending downward (see Figure 11.21 on p. 231). Her delivery of DTI reflected Data Profile A, and so, following the appropriate action steps, implementation and data collection continued. However, her delivery of the BSP reflected Data Profile C and so, following the appropriate action steps, an implementation support needed to be identified and provided. Ms. Smith documented evaluating the intervention on the Implementation Tracking Log (see Figure 11.2).

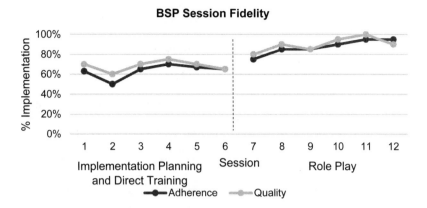

FIGURE 11.19. Ms. Davis's intervention fidelity data after role play.

Step 10: Support Implementation

MS. LEE: PERFORMANCE-BUILDING IMPLEMENTATION SUPPORT— PERFORMANCE FEEDBACK

Although initially Ms. Lee demonstrated a skill deficit (i.e., did not implement some steps of the plan, implemented with low levels of quality), following participant modeling her data aligned more with a performance deficit in that she implemented BSP and DTI intervention steps with some variability (65–90%), but could demonstrate fluent implementation with high quality for all steps and had been observed to implement all steps with adequate adherence. Therefore, Ms. Smith decided it would be appropriate to provide Ms. Lee with regular performance feedback until implementation increased to desired levels across time (i.e., above 80% consistently).

Before meeting with Ms. Lee, Ms. Smith reviewed the intervention and current data, read about performance feedback, scheduled the performance feedback session, and gath-

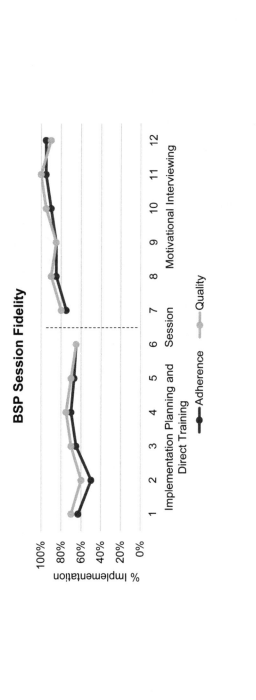

BSP Session Fidelity

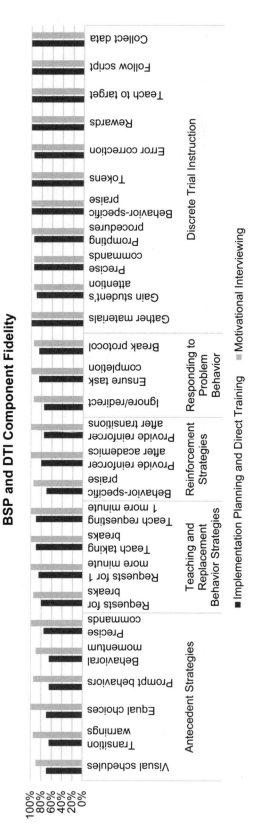

BSP and DTI Component Fidelity

■ Implementation Planning and Direct Training   ■ Motivational Interviewing

FIGURE 11.20. Ms. Garcia's intervention fidelity data after motivational interviewing.

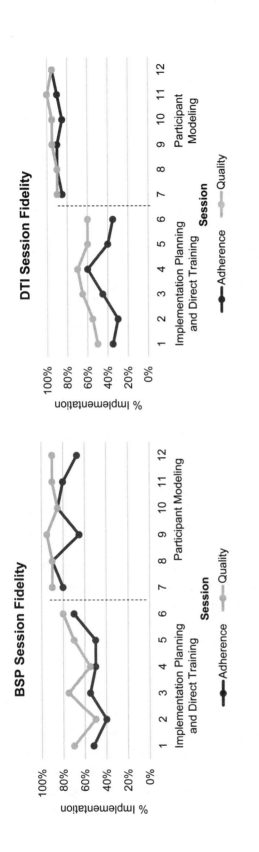

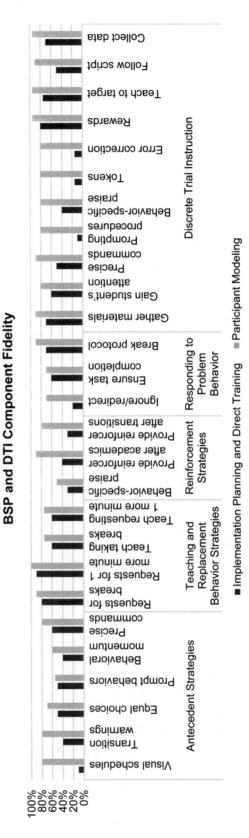

FIGURE 11.21. Ms. Lee's intervention fidelity data after participant modeling.

231

ered session materials. Ms. Smith also prepared learner and implementation graphs to share with Ms. Lee and scheduled a meeting with her. At the meeting, Ms. Smith first explained the purpose of the meeting (Step 1) and then asked for Ms. Lee's perspective on the BSP implementation and learner progress (Steps 2 and 3). Ms. Lee answered: "I think things are going OK. I feel a lot more comfortable with providing the plan as a whole since you and Mr. Hall worked with me a few weeks ago. I think sometimes I still struggle with providing enough prevention strategies, and I tend to lean on the responsive procedures—which I know isn't the point of the plan. The academic lessons have been going really well, though. Kyle has made great strides with letter naming and counting objects—we're really excited about that. I think his behavior during academic times has been a bit better too, but the transitions from preferred activities are still a struggle."

Ms. Smith then reviewed the intervention fidelity data with Ms. Lee (Step 4), noting the steps that she consistently implemented with high levels of adherence and quality (e.g., using a within-task schedule, providing transition warnings, following criteria to prompt a break) and the steps that were more challenging for her to consistently implement (e.g., prompting replacement behaviors, using high rates of behavior-specific praise). Similarly, Ms. Smith reviewed the morning learner outcome data (Step 5) and highlighted that although Kyle was making some progress, it was likely that increases in intervention fidelity would lead to greater gains in learner outcomes. Ms. Smith and Ms. Lee reviewed and practiced the steps identified as being implemented inconsistently and then problem-solved ways to improve implementation (Step 6). Ms. Lee thought that adding additional prompts, such as visuals, Post-it Notes, and a cuing device, would help her remember to implement interventions more consistently (Step 7). They set a goal for 87% or greater adherence (i.e., steps that were implemented as planned) for the week, based on her current level of 77%. They also discussed that is was important to decrease the variability in the data so that she had more days on which her consistency was at or above 80% implementation, whereas her current data ranged from 60 to 100%. They decided it would be helpful to meet on a weekly basis to provide ongoing performance feedback until Ms. Lee had reached her implementation goals, and that she should write down any questions she had while implementing to be reviewed at these meeting. Ms. Smith thanked Ms. Lee for participating in performance feedback (Step 8). Ms. Smith also completed the corresponding Fidelity Data Sheet for Direct Training (Appendix 10.2) to note that Ms. Lee had received this support as planned, and she documented the provision of this support on the Implementation Tracking Log (see Figure 11.2).

After three performance feedback sessions, Ms. Lee met her implementation goal (see Figure 11.22). Upon further review of the learner outcome and intervention fidelity data, each implementer was demonstrating consistently high levels of adherence and quality, both for the BSP and DTI lessons. Learner outcomes were on track to meet goals at school and at home (see Figures 11.23 and 11.18). Data Profile A had been achieved, the interventions were continued, implementation data collection was continued, but the frequency of collection was reduced and transferred largely to the self-report format because the implementers were found to be accurate raters, and the data were reviewed on a biweekly basis to ensure that progress maintained.

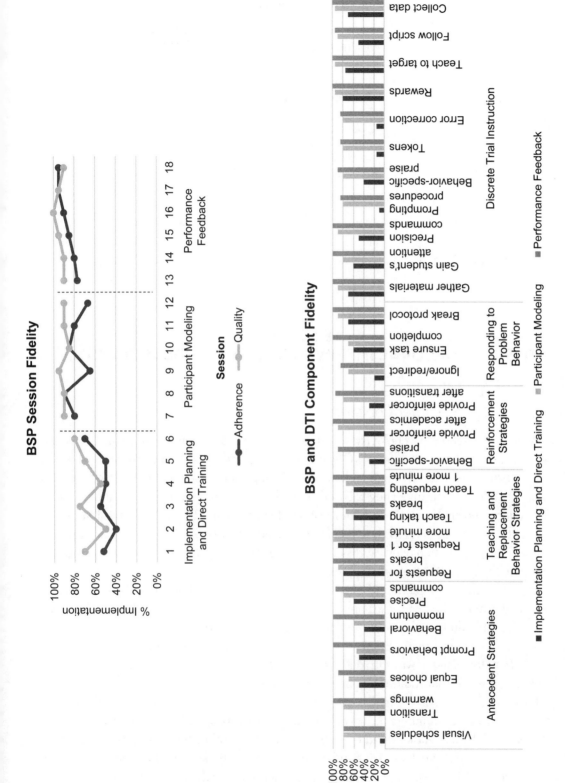

FIGURE 11.22. Ms. Lee's intervention fidelity after participant modeling and performance feedback.

233

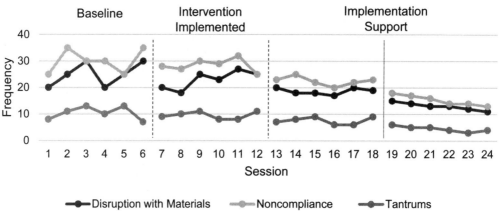

FIGURE 11.23. Learner outcomes after all implementation supports provided.

CASE STUDY 2:
TIER 2 BEHAVIORAL INTERVENTION IN A MIDDLE SCHOOL

Phase 1: Prepare

Step 1: Identify a Learner Concern

Mr. Wilson, the school psychologist, and the seventh-grade teachers on Team "A" began reviewing office discipline referral (ODR) data and grades, discussing students who had been struggling behaviorally and academically, during their biweekly multi-tiered systems of support (MTSS) meeting. They focused on discussing three students (Anthony, Gloria, and Xander) who had met the school's criteria for receiving Tier 2 behavioral supports based on the number of ODRs they received. Teacher reports confirmed that the students displayed "disruptive behavior" across classes (see Figure 11.24) and that these students would benefit from intervention. The teachers reported that students' disruptive behavior was impeding their completion of classwork, which negatively impacted their grades. At times the disruptive behavior escalated to the point where the students raised their voices when talking to adults and failed to comply with adult directives. This behavior has been occurring more frequently within the last few weeks, which was supported by ODR data.

Additionally, Xander was currently struggling academically in math. Ms. Blake, the math teacher, noted that Xander had been performing around the class average all year but was doing poorly with solving multistep, real-life, and mathematical problems with positive and negative rational numbers (i.e., whole numbers, fractions, and decimals; CCS.MATH.CONTENT.7.EE.B.3). Xander had done fine with solving other types of application problems in math this year, such as ratios and geometry, so Ms. Blake hypothesized that Xander was struggling with the specific calculations and not necessarily the word-problem format. When Ms. Blake further evaluated Xander's permanent products, she noted that the questions he consistently got wrong involved negative rational numbers. Anecdotally, Ms. Blake

Stakeholders	

Team:
 • School psychologist, Mr. Wilson
 • "Team A" seventh-grade teachers
   o English teacher, Mr. Rodriguez
   o Math teacher, Ms. Blake
   o Science teacher, Ms. Garcia
   o History teacher, Mr. Sullivan
 • CICO coordinator, Ms. Morales
	Learners: Seventh-grade general education students on "Team A"
	 • Anthony
	 • Gloria
	 • Xander

Learner Concerns	

Behavior Concerns—Anthony, Gloria, and Xander:
 • *Disruptive behavior:* Any instance of behavior that interrupts or distracts from learning.
   o *Examples:* Calling out answers, talking about nonacademic subjects with peers, walking around the room, and using materials not needed for assignments.
   o *Non-examples:* Talking to peers about work-related topics during a group activity, responding to teacher questions using an appropriate tone/content.
 	
 Academic Concerns—Xander: Math accuracy in the skill area of solving calculations involving negative rational numbers in any form (whole numbers, fractions, and decimals).	

FIGURE 11.24. Case study 2 overview.

noticed that Xander moved through these problems slowly as well. After the meeting, Mr. Wilson documented the completion of this step on the Implementation Tracking Log (see Figure 11.25 on pp. 236–237).

Step 2: Collect Baseline Data

The team decided to take a closer look at and monitor extant data sources, such as grades and ODRs, and collect some additional information. Based on the presenting student concerns and availability of Tier 2 interventions, the team decided that if the data indicated a need to intervene, they would begin a check-in/check-out (CICO) intervention (described in Step 4) to support student behavior. At the end of each class period, teachers rated student behavior on a 0- to 2-point scale, based on how well students followed each of the school-wide behavioral expectations (i.e., safe, responsible, respectful; see Figure 11.26 on p. 238). Students did not know that teachers were collecting data on their behaviors during the baseline phase, and therefore the ratings were not shared. Data were entered into an Excel spreadsheet by Mr. Wilson and graphed according to time period and expectation.

To further assess Xander's math difficulties and determine specific areas of deficit for computation, Ms. Blake administered 2-minute curriculum-based measurement (CBM) probes related to computation problems for negative rational numbers (i.e., addition, subtraction, multiplication, division of whole numbers, fractions, and decimals). Mr. Wilson scored all CBM probes for accuracy and fluency and documented the completion of this step on the Implementation Tracking Log (see Figure 11.25).

Learner: _Anthony, Gloria, Xander_   Implementers: _"Team A" seventh-grade teachers (Mr. Rodriguez, Ms. Blake, Ms. Garcia, Mr. Sullivan), CICO coordinator (Ms. Morales)_

Consultant: _Mr. Wilson_   Intervention: _CICO (all), math fluency intervention (Xander)_

Use this worksheet to document the implementation process.

Date	Activity/Meeting	Action Steps	Person Responsible	Date Due	Notes
Phase 1: Prepare					
11/3	1. Identify learner concerns	• Conduct team meeting to operationalize concerns • Plan to collect baseline data	Consultant Consultant	11/5	
11/5	2. Collect baseline data	• Collect behavior data (CICO form) • Collect CBM math data • Summarize baseline data	"Team A" teachers Ms. Blake Consultant	11/20	
11/20	3. Confirm the concern and set a goal	• Decide if there is a concern to be addressed • Develop SMART goals	Consultant and school-based team Consultant	11/22	
11/22	4. Identify the intervention	• Obtain intervention materials • Develop a draft of intervention fidelity materials	Consultant, CICO coordinator Consultant	12/1	
12/1	5. Planfully adapt the intervention to the context/resources (i.e., provide implementation planning)	• Share the implementation plan	Consultant	12/5	
12/1	6. Provide high-quality training	• Train the implementers • Make sure the intervention materials are available to the implementers	Consultant, CICO coordinator Consultant, CICO coordinator	12/5	

FIGURE 11.25. Case study 2 Implementation Tracking Log.

(continued)

236

Date	Activity/Meeting	Action Steps	Person Responsible	Date Due	Notes
Phase 2: Implement and Evaluate					
12/5	7. Implement the intervention	• Determine dates for implementation and learner outcome assessment	Implementers	11/10	
12/5	8a. Collect learner outcome data	• Graph the data • Interpret the data	CICO coordinator, Ms. Blake Consultant	1/3	
12/5	8b. Collect intervention fidelity data	• Graph and interpret the data • Develop a summary statement	Consultant Consultant	1/3	
1/3	9. Evaluate the intervention and make data-based decisions (use Data-Based Decision-Making Worksheet)	• Identify action steps based on the data profile	Consultant	1/5	
Phase 3: Support (as needed)					
1/5	10. Support implementation	• Provide self-monitoring support to Ms. Blake and a copy of a self-monitoring form • Revise the implementation plan with Ms. Morales and provide a copy of the updated plan • Enact role playing with Mr. Rodriguez	Consultant Consultant Consultant	1/15	
1/15	11. Evaluate the intervention	• Evaluate intervention fidelity and learner outcome data	Consultant	2/5	

FIGURE 11.25. (*(continued)*)

Student: _____ Date: _____

Your teacher will complete ratings at the end of each period. Bring this form with you to Ms. Morales at the end of the day.

Key: 2 = independent (two or fewer reminders needed), 1 = some support (three to five reminders needed), 0 = significant support (six or more reminders needed)

	Teacher Initials	Respectful • Work quietly • Raise hand and wait to be called on • Use respectful language • Focus on self			Responsible • Be on time with materials • Ask for help when you need it • Complete work and use time management			Safe • Stay in your seat • Keep hands and feet to yourself • Maintain personal space • Use classroom materials appropriately		
Period 1		0	1	2	0	1	2	0	1	2
Period 2		0	1	2	0	1	2	0	1	2
Period 3		0	1	2	0	1	2	0	1	2
Period 4		0	1	2	0	1	2	0	1	2
Period 5		0	1	2	0	1	2	0	1	2
Period 6		0	1	2	0	1	2	0	1	2
Period 7		0	1	2	0	1	2	0	1	2
Total Points		_____/14			_____/14			_____/14		
		Overall Points: _____/42		Today's %: _____			Goal %: _____			

FIGURE 11.26. CICO point sheet.

Step 3: Confirm the Concern and Set a Goal

After data were gathered for 1 week, the team came together to review the summarized data (see Figure 11.27). Overall, Anthony was earning an average of 60% of possible points for following behavioral expectations, Gloria was earning 70% of points, and Xander was earning 65% of points. During CBM probes, on average, Xander was also only correctly solving 40% of math calculations involving negative rational numbers. The team collaborated to write SMART goals based on each student's baseline data (see Figure 11.28). Mr. Wilson documented the completion of this step on the Implementation Tracking Log (see Figure 11.25).

Step 4: Identify an Intervention

The team agreed that based on the typography of the behavior and its consistency across settings, as well as the observation that the students enjoyed and responded well to adult attention, a CICO intervention would be a good fit for each student and feasible for the teachers to implement (see Figure 11.29). The plan was that Ms. Morales, the CICO coordinator (and art teacher), would meet with the students briefly (< 5 minutes) each morning and afternoon. In the morning, she would give the students with a new point sheet, make sure that they had all materials needed to be successful in class, and encourage them to make their behavioral goal by being safe, responsible, and respectful in class. During each class period, teachers

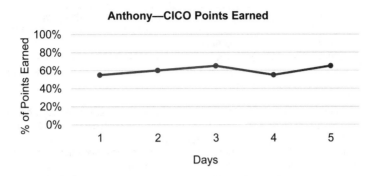

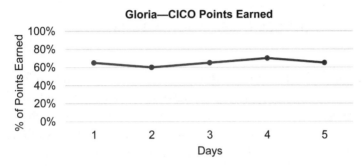

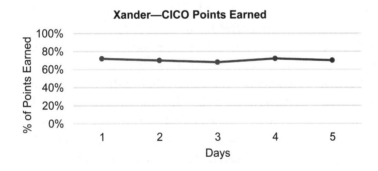

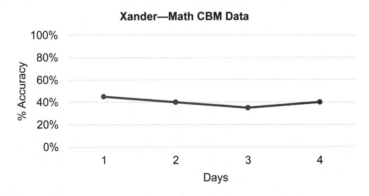

FIGURE 11.27. Learner baseline data.

- *Anthony*: Given consistent feedback on behavior and contingent rewards, Anthony will increase his CICO points earned from 60 to 80% over a 2-month period and maintain this increase across 80% of days over a 2-week period before increasing his goal percentage further.
- *Gloria*: Given consistent feedback on behavior and contingent rewards, Gloria will increase her CICO points earned from 70 to 90% over a 2-month period and maintain this increase across 80% of days over a 2-week period before transitioning to a CICO self-monitoring intervention.
- *Xander*:
  - Given consistent feedback on behavior and contingent rewards, Xander will increase his CICO points earned from 65 to 85% over a 2-month period and maintain this increase across 80% of days over a 2-week period before increasing his goal percentage further.
  - Given daily practice and feedback on math calculations involving negative rational numbers, Xander will increase his math accuracy from 40 to 80% over a 2-month period.

FIGURE 11.28. Case study 2 SMART goals.

would prompt expected behaviors at the beginning of the class and offer encouragement, provide behavior-specific praise for target behaviors occurring throughout the class period, calmly remind students of expected behavior whenever they made behavioral errors, rate the students' behavior on the CICO form during the last 5 minutes of class, and provide specific feedback to the students about their behavior, using a praise–correct–praise format. Students would bring the point sheet with them to each class period, but teachers had extra copies in case students lost theirs. At the end of the day, students would again meet with Ms. Morales to discuss the positives and areas to improve for the day and total the points with the students to check if the their overall percentage of points earned met their daily goal. Daily goals would be set at 5% above baseline and increase by 5% each time a student earned two rewards for that goal level. Students would chart their individual progress on a graph and mark checks on a progress chart for each day they met their goals. Students would earn a reward for meeting their goals on four nonconsecutive days. Ms. Morales would record when students earned a reward on a data-tracking sheet. Reward options would be identified for students based on the results of a preference assessment; students would select the reward they were working toward when they begin CICO and choose a new reward to work toward during morning check-in the day after they had earned a reward.

- Intervention provided daily.
- *Check-in:* The CICO coordinator meets with students briefly (< 5 minutes) in her office to distribute the point sheets, make sure they have all materials needed to be successful in class, and encourage them to make their behavioral goal by being respectful, responsible, and safe in class.
- *During each class period:* Teachers prompt expected behaviors at the beginning of the class period and offer encouragement, provide behavior-specific praise for target behaviors throughout the class period, calmly remind students of expected behavior when students make behavioral errors, rate students' behavior on the CICO forms during the last 5 minutes of class, and provide specific feedback to students about their behavior, using a praise–correct–praise format.
- *Check-out:* The CICO coordinator meets with students briefly (< 10 minutes) to discuss the positive accomplishments, the areas to improve for the day, and the total points earned to determine if students met their daily goals. Students chart their individual progress on a graph and make a checkmark on a progress chart for each day that they met their goals. A reward is provided when students meet their goals on four nonconsecutive days.

FIGURE 11.29. Case study 2 CICO intervention plan.

- Computer-assisted instruction that provides immediate visual corrective feedback on accurately solving computation problems for negative rational numbers provided daily for 15 minutes during Xander's study skills block.
- Small reward contingent on earning a certain number of points in a session.

FIGURE 11.30. Math intervention overview.

The team members also decided that Xander would benefit from a math accuracy intervention. They decided on a computer-assisted instruction program that provided immediate visual corrective feedback for accurately solving computation problems involving negative rational numbers (see Figure 11.30). Xander would earn points for typing correct responses. If he typed the answer incorrectly, he would not earn points, the answer would show up on the screen, and he had to type in the correct answer three times before moving on. This program includes opportunities to practice skills (e.g., addition, subtraction, multiplication, division) for different types of rational numbers (e.g., whole numbers, fractions, decimals) in isolation before meeting mastery criteria and moving on to the next skill. If Xander earned a predetermined number of points in a session, he would earn a reward, delivered by Ms. Blake. The program automatically records data so the teacher can track a student's progress. Xander would receive this intervention in Ms. Blake's room for 15 minutes each day during a study skills block.

The team shared the intervention plans with each student's family and received permission to begin Tier 2 supports before beginning implementation. Mr. Wilson documented the completion of Step 4, "Identify the Intervention," on the Implementation Tracking Log (see Figure 11.25).

Step 5: Planfully Adapt the Intervention to the Context/Resources

After the behavioral and academic interventions were identified, the team reconvened to engage in a proactive process of implementation support and planning. During this process, the team had a chance to planfully adapt intervention components to the specific context, embed the implementer's preferences, and document these modifications. Before meeting with the team, Mr. Wilson reviewed the intervention, broke down the intervention plan into concrete steps, read about implementation planning, prepared action and coping planning worksheets, and practiced the dialogue. During the meeting, Mr. Wilson first explained the purpose of implementation planning (Step 1), reviewed the target concerns and goals (Step 2), and reviewed the intervention steps (Step 3). The team decided not to modify any of the intervention steps, as they found both interventions to be feasible and acceptable (Step 4). However, they did clarify that (a) a preference assessment needed to be completed for each student, (b) Ms. Morales would provide the students with an orientation to the CICO program, (c) Ms. Morales would enter data and determine when students earned rewards and could increase goal percentages based on set criteria, and (d) Ms. Blake would talk to Xander about using the first 15 minutes of her study skills time to participate in the math intervention. The team then participated in action planning for both the CICO and math interventions, during which they identified logistics for each intervention step (Step

5; when, how often, for how long, where, resources needed) and how resources, such as rewards and CICO forms, would be obtained (Step 6). Mr. Wilson then summarized the action plan (Step 7), before moving on to coping planning. During coping planning, the team identified possible barriers to consistently delivering the intervention (Step 8) and brainstormed strategies to address the barriers (Step 9). Mr. Wilson then summarized the coping plan (Step 10) and thanked the team for meeting with him and thinking through the details of implementing the intervention (Step 11). He provided the team with a clean copy of the implementation plan within the week, documented the provision of this step on the Implementation Tracking Log (see Figure 11.25), and completed the Fidelity Data Sheet for Implementation Planning (Appendix 5.3). The action and coping plans for the CICO and math interventions are provided in Figure 11.31.

Step 6: Provide High-Quality Training

Each teacher had previously received a training session on CICO as part of the schoolwide rollout of the Tier 2 intervention. However, they had not yet implemented the intervention during the current school year, so they agreed that they could benefit from a booster training. They watched a training video, created by members of the MTSS committee, which demonstrated the essential components of CICO in the classroom. They also had an opportunity to ask questions about and practice the intervention with Mr. Wilson, who gave them feedback after their practice. Mr. Wilson documented this step on the Implementation Tracking Log (see Figure 11.25).

Additionally, Ms. Blake had already used this computerized math intervention with students in the past and felt comfortable with facilitating the delivery of the intervention and analyzing the reported data. No additional training occurred, as the intervention was provided on the computer, which eliminated implementation errors. The only foreseeable issue would be making sure that Xander came to Ms. Blake's room at the correct time daily and engaged with the program for 15 minutes.

Phase 2: Implement and Evaluate

Step 7: Implement the Intervention

After logistical details were finalized and training was provided, the team initiated implementation of the behavioral and academic interventions, which were documented on the Implementation Tracking Log (see Figure 11.25).

Step 8a: Assess Learner Outcomes

The team recognized that one of the major benefits of the CICO intervention was that the points and feedback not only served to support student behavior, but also acted as a data collection system. Therefore, the team could easily monitor the percentage of points each student earned. They could evaluate these data in relation to behavioral expectation and setting. They could also evaluate how frequently the student met his or her goal and earned rewards.

Action Plan: CICO					
Intervention Step	**To Be Implemented**				**Resources Needed?**
	When?	**How Often?**	**For How Long?**	**Where?**	
Conduct preference assessment	Before starting CICO intervention	Once for formal paired-choice assessment and then informally after student reaches goal and selects new reward	15 minutes	CICO coordinator's office	Preference assessment form; ensure consistent access to rewards
Orient students to CICO	Before starting CICO intervention	Once	15 minutes	CICO coordinator's office	Point sheet, schoolwide behavioral expectations matrix, graph paper to practice charting points
Check in	CICO room open during last 15 minutes of morning flex time before Period 1	Daily	< 5 minutes per student	CICO coordinator's office	Point sheet, pencils, pens, and other academic materials in case students need them
Prompt behavioral expectations	At the beginning of and throughout class	Before each new activity at a minimum	Takes < 1 minute each time	Throughout classroom	N/A
Provide behavior-specific praise	During each class	Every time a student engages in expected behavior	Takes < 1 minute each time	Throughout classroom	N/A
Calmly provide error corrections	During class	When student engages in problem behavior that does not respond to planned ignoring or other strategies	Takes < 1 minute each time	Throughout classroom	N/A
Provide feedback on points	Last 5 minutes of class	Once per class	Takes < 2 minutes per student	At teacher's desk	Point sheet
Check out	During last 10 minutes of Period 7	Each day	Takes < 5 minutes per student	CICO coordinator's office	Point sheet, point tracking sheet, graph paper
Provide reward	During lunch, study skills block, or check-out time, depending on what student has chosen— within a day of meeting criteria	When student has met his or her goal on four nonconsecutive days	Depends on what reward student has chosen—a tangible, edible, or homework pass (< 3 minutes), playing a game with peers or staff (~15 minutes), etc.	Varies by reward	Varies by reward
Monitor and enter data	After school	Biweekly	Takes < 10 minutes per student	CICO coordinator's office	Computer, point sheets

(continued)

FIGURE 11.31. Case study 2 action and coping plans.

Coping Plan: CICO	
Potential Major Barrier to Intervention Implementation	**Strategy to Implement the Intervention Nevertheless**
Student forgets to come to check-in or check-out time	Provide reminders/incentives for coming to CICO time; allow student to bring friend with him or her
Student does not meet goal points	Examine level of implementation fidelity; reassess student preferences
CICO coordinator or teacher absent	A trained "backup" CICO coordinator is available; develop a "cheat sheet" about CICO to leave with substitute teachers
Student does not bring CICO form to class	Provide additional forms; if chronic issue, consider having teachers enter data at the end of each period directly into a shared spreadsheet and show the student these data

Action Plan: Math Intervention					
Intervention Step	**To Be Implemented**				**Resources Needed?**
	When?	**How Often?**	**For How Long?**	**Where?**	
Computer-assisted instruction	First part of study skills	Daily	15 minutes	Ms. Blake's classroom	Computer
Contingent reward	Points checked after 15-minute session completed	When student earns certain number of points during instruction	Reward (e.g., food, tangible) given quickly	Ms. Blake's classroom	Rewards

Coping Plan: Math Intervention	
Potential Major Barrier to Intervention Implementation	**Strategy to Implement the Intervention Nevertheless**
Ms. Blake is busy during study skills period, and it may be challenging for her to consistently log Xander on to the computer	Teach Xander to independently log on to the computer program so he does not need Ms. Blake's help

FIGURE 11.31. *(continued)*

In addition to the data collected on the computer-delivered math intervention, Ms. Blake would administer CBM math probes to Xander on a twice-weekly basis. The team also decided that ODR and grade data would continue to provide important supplementary information that they would review during treatment evaluation, but this did not require any extra data collection effort. The team documented these steps on the Implementation Tracking Log (see Figure 11.25).

Step 8b: Assess Intervention Fidelity

Intervention fidelity data were also collected. Mr. Wilson first considered the intensiveness of the intervention and possible decisions that might result from a lack of student response. Both the academic and behavioral interventions were considered Tier 2 interventions, as they were standardized and systematized (i.e., multiple students could receive the same protocol), and were fairly resource efficient. If students did not respond, the interventions would be adapted or intensified, but at this point the students were not in danger of serious disciplinary actions or being referred for a special education assessment. However, the interventions were clearly more intense than Tier 1 interventions. Mr. Wilson considered multiple methods of intervention fidelity data collection (see Figure 11.32). Using permanent products was an obvious option, as rating could easily be provided if teachers gave students points or not. However, this method would not capture if a teacher provided (1) intervention steps throughout the period, such as prompting and praise; and (2) appropriate feedback to the student at the end of class, or just circled a number on the point sheet. Given the number of students on CICO, however, Mr. Wilson decided that it was not feasible to regularly conduct direction observations of implementation, but that he could spot-check implementation adherence by conducting a direct observation during one class for each implementer every 2 weeks.

Classroom teachers rated their implementation of CICO components daily during one class period—a period that was on a rotating schedule, as the target students were in different classes. Teachers rated themselves immediately after the class was over to promote accurate reporting. The rating form listed specific intervention steps, such as prompted, praised, and provided feedback, and asked teachers to rate their adherence to each step on a 0- to 2-point scale. Mr. Wilson collected the forms weekly to summarize and graph. He used the same form when collecting his implementation checks. Similarly, Ms. Morales completed daily CICO implementation checklists for each student in the CICO program, thereby documenting if students attended check-in and check-out times as a measure of exposure, and if she completed each relevant step on the implementation plan, as a measure of her adherence.

Mr. Wilson collected the completed CICO forms from Ms. Morales at the end of the week and rated the permanent products using a checklist. He summarized the percentage of ratings completed by each teacher over the week.

Finally, for Xander's academic intervention, the computer program not only provided progress reports, but also logged how long a student was using the intervention. The duration information was a measure of exposure and could be compared to the number of minutes that Xander was scheduled to receive the intervention per week. The collection of learner outcome and intervention fidelity data was documented on the Implementation Tracking Log (see Figure 11.25).

Direct Observation
- Mr. Wilson observes each teacher implementing the intervention for one class every other week.
- Likert scale (0–2) data tracks adherence to CICO components implemented in the classroom.

Self-Report
- Classroom teachers complete a once-daily Likert scale (0–2) rating on their adherence to implementing CICO components during one class period.
- Ms. Morales (CICO coordinator) completes daily checklists for each student in the CICO program, including students' attendance at CICO times and their completion of CICO steps from the implementation plan.

Permanent Product
- Mr. Wilson rates CICO forms for completion using a yes/no checklist and summarizes the percentage of ratings completed by each teacher over a week.
- The math program automatically records the duration of Xander's time using the program, which in turn provides a measure of adherence and exposure to the intervention.

FIGURE 11.32. Case study 2 intervention fidelity data collection plan.

Step 9: Evaluate the Intervention and Make a Data-Based Decision

Learner outcome and intervention fidelity data were entered into a database, graphed, and visually analyzed on a weekly basis. After 1 month of implementation, Mr. Wilson summarized the intervention fidelity data (permanent product, self-report, and direct observation) by overall implementation level. He reviewed the level, trend, and variability of the data to decide whether the interventions were delivered to the extent that it could be reasonably expected that the learners would benefit. The following sections describe the intervention fidelity data, learner outcomes, and next steps based on the evaluation of these two data sources.

INTERVENTION FIDELITY DATA

• Intervention fidelity generally did not vary based on the student to whom the implementer was providing CICO. Therefore, an aggregate of adherence is provided across students for each implementer and exceptions are noted.

• Mr. Rodriguez (English teacher) inconsistently completed the CICO form across students (a rating was provided only 60% of the time). He was an accurate self-reporter and acknowledged when he did not complete the ratings or provide feedback to students. Self-report and direct observation data did indicate that he provided high rates of praise to target students (and his classes in general), but he did not prompt behavioral expectations at the beginning of class (ratings of "0"). See Figure 11.33 for his intervention fidelity data.

• Ms. Blake (math teacher) demonstrated variable implementation of the CICO intervention across students (see Figure 11.34 on p. 248). Although she consistently completed point sheets (i.e., 90% of days), she acknowledged that she did not always provide students with complete feedback about their behavior and points earned as outlined in the intervention (i.e., praise–correct–praise). She also did not consistently provide high levels of praise to the target students throughout the entire class period. Further, Mr. Wilson noticed that Xander had not completed the correct dosage of math intervention. He had only logged on for an average of 5 minutes per day, instead of the 15 minutes per day written in his plan. Mr. Wilson would need to follow up with Ms. Blake about possible reasons why Xander was not completing the intervention for the full 15 minutes.

• Ms. Garcia (science teacher) consistently prompted, praised, and provided appropriate error corrections to her students (average: 90% of the time). During the first 2 weeks of implementation, she completed all CICO forms for all students except Gloria. When Mr. Wilson checked in with Ms. Garcia about this, she reported that Gloria has her class right after lunch and often does not have her CICO form. Mr. Wilson reminded Ms. Garcia to provide Gloria with a new CICO form. However, Mr. Wilson talked to the rest of the team and found out that Gloria inconsistently brought her form to class periods after lunch, which negatively impacted his point totals. Because of this, a change was made: Gloria now had a point sheet that she left with the teacher whose class she had before lunch and who put it in Ms. Morales's mailbox, and in turn received a new point sheet for after lunch in Ms. Garcia's classroom, which she brought with her for the rest of the day, to check-out. After this change, Ms. Garcia rated Gloria's behavior with a high level of adherence (see Figure 11.35 on p. 249).

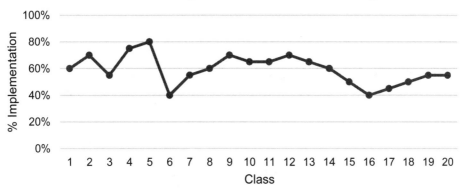

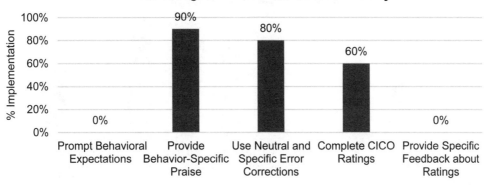

FIGURE 11.33. Mr. Rodriguez's CICO intervention fidelity data after direct training and implementation planning.

• Mr. Sullivan implemented the CICO intervention with 90% adherence across students and steps (see Figure 11.36 on p. 250).

• Ms. Morales implemented all steps of the check-in and check-out process consistently for each student (see Figure 11.37 on p. 251). Her data also indicated that students were regularly attending these brief meetings, so exposure was not an issue. However, Mr. Wilson did notice that Ms. Morales's data-tracking form indicated that rewards were not provided immediately after students met criteria to receive them and were typically delayed by 2 days.

LEARNER DATA

For a visual representation of learner data, refer to Figure 11.38 (p. 252).

• Anthony was making sufficient progress toward his goal of earning 80% of his points in 2 months. In 1 month, he had increased his average to 70% of points.

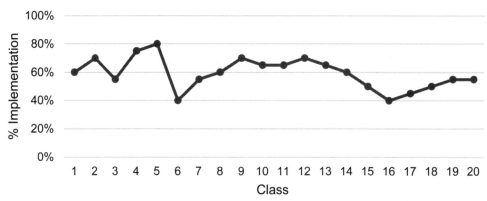

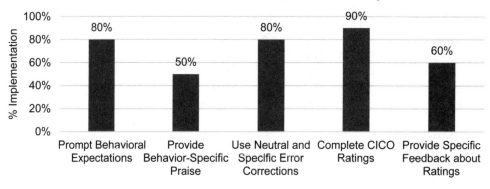

FIGURE 11.34. Ms. Blake's CICO intervention fidelity data after direct training and implementation planning.

• Gloria was making insufficient progress toward her goal of earning 90% of her points in 2 months. After 1 month of CICO, Gloria's average points earned had increased only to 75%.

• Xander was making insufficient progress toward his behavioral goal of earning 85% of points in 2 months. His average points earned increased from 65 to 70% in the month since beginning implementation, and it was highly variable. Additionally, Xander had only increased his math accuracy to 55%, whereas at this point in time, he should have attained 65%.

Based on these data, Anthony was on track to meet his goals despite insufficient intervention fidelity. This aligns with Data Profile B. The team decided to update his intervention goal to 85% of points earned and support intervention fidelity. The team also discovered that Anthony's mom had made copies of the point sheet that was sent home when asking for permission to participate in the intervention, and she started using it with Anthony after school to promote his appropriate behavior when asked to complete chores and homework. She also tied the points to rewards, so the team hypothesized that receiving the intervention in an addition setting was supporting Anthony's response to the intervention at school.

Gloria (CICO) and Xander (CICO and math intervention) were not on track to meet their intervention goals, and the intervention fidelity data for their respective interventions were insufficient. This summary fits with Data Profile C. The various implementers needed implementation support based on their specific difficulties with implementation.

• Mr. Rodriguez did not deliver some of the intervention steps (e.g., prompting behavioral expectations). Mr. Wilson considered implementation supports to address this skill deficit.

• Ms. Blake displayed variable adherence. She had demonstrated the ability to implement all intervention steps but did so inconsistently. Further, Xander was not being exposed to the math intervention for the entire 15 minutes daily. Mr. Wilson reviewed the imple-

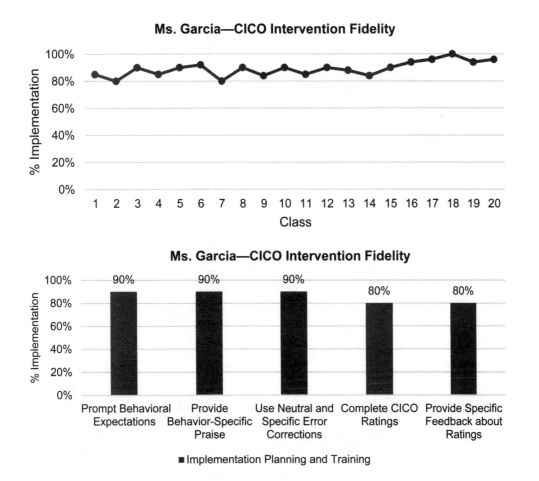

FIGURE 11.35. Ms. Garcia's CICO intervention fidelity data after direct training and implementation planning.

mentation support options for performance deficits and made a note to discuss and problem-solve additional barriers that were impeding her consistent implementation of the math intervention.

• Ms. Garcia and Mr. Sullivan demonstrated consistently high levels of implementation. Data by time of day also indicated that the students receiving intervention were more likely to have successful days behaviorally in their classrooms. Therefore, their intervention fidelity data will be regularly monitored and implementation supports provided only if data indicate a need in the future.

• Ms. Morales implemented all CICO steps correctly but was having difficulty consistently delivering rewards to students immediately when they were earned. Mr. Wilson reviewed the implementation support options he could provide to address this performance deficit.

The process for each implementer was documented on the Implementation Tracking Log (see Figure 11.25).

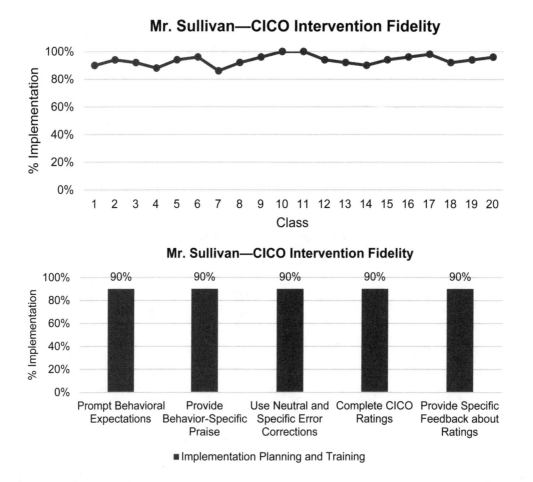

FIGURE 11.36. Mr. Sullivan's CICO intervention fidelity data after direct training and implementation planning.

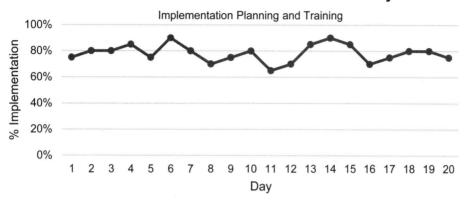

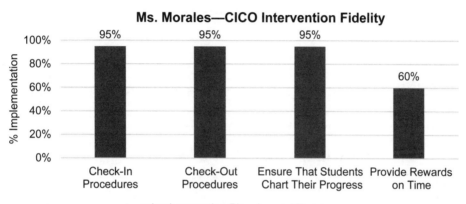

FIGURE 11.37. Ms. Morales's CICO intervention fidelity data after direct training and implementation planning.

Phase 3: Support

Step 10: Support Implementation

Based on the intervention fidelity data, Ms. Blake, Ms. Morales, and Mr. Rodriguez required additional implementation support.

MS. BLAKE: PERFORMANCE-BUILDING IMPLEMENTATION SUPPORT—
SELF-MONITORING

Ms. Blake's implementation difficulties were related to performance deficits with implementing the CICO intervention. Ms. Blake was an accurate self-reporter and was invested in collecting accurate data for the students with whom she worked. To incorporate these implementer preferences and strengths and provide a way for Ms. Blake to hold herself accountable for delivering certain steps of the CICO intervention (i.e., consistently providing praise and feedback), Mr. Wilson decided to support her implementation by teaching

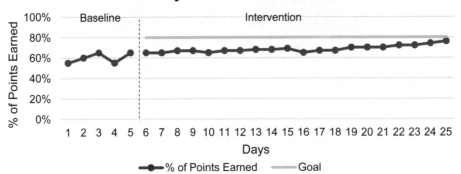

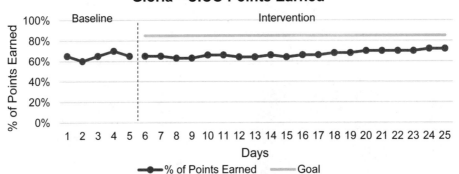

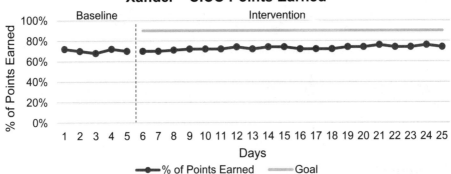

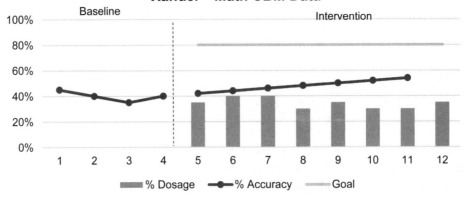

FIGURE 11.38. Learner data after intervention.

her self-monitoring. Before meeting with Ms. Blake, Mr. Wilson reviewed the intervention form and self-report data collection form, reviewed the current data, read about self-monitoring, brainstormed some possible ways Ms. Blake could self-monitor, and scheduled the meeting. Mr. Wilson first reviewed the purpose of the meeting, highlighting learner outcomes and providing an overview of why self-monitoring works to promote implementation (Step 1). Next he described the rationale for implementing each intervention step, reviewed how to implement each intervention step, and reviewed the corresponding intervention step fidelity data (Step 2). He highlighted the areas that Ms. Blake was consistently implementing and where she might benefit from self-monitoring. Mr. Wilson then transitioned to discussing what the self-monitoring tool might look like (Step 3). He had drafted a form with a space for Ms. Blake to tally her praise statements to the target students as well as a more specific checklist of feedback steps than the general "provided feedback." These items were both embedded into the original self-report form. Ms. Blake liked the idea of recording the number of praise statements she gave to each target student, but thought doing so during three full class periods would be too much, so she tallied during 15 minutes of each class period. Mr. Wilson modeled how Ms. Wilson would use the forms to self-monitor and gave her an opportunity to practice (Step 4). They then discussed possible adaptations to self-monitoring (Step 5). Ms. Wilson liked the idea of self-evaluation. They decided that she would summarize and graph her implementation data each week. They also set a goal of 80% implementation for the intervention steps she was inconsistently implementing and would set an additional goal for increasing the number of praise statements provided after data were collected for a few days. Mr. Wilson clarified the self-monitoring data collection plan: Every day during one class period, Ms. Blake would continue to collect self-report data with the more specific feedback steps and tally praise frequency data for 15 minutes. Ms. Black would continue to rotate the class in which she collected data (Step 6). Mr. Wilson thanked Ms. Blake for her willingness to try self-monitoring (Step 7).

Mr. Wilson then reviewed the data on the amount of time Xander was receiving his math intervention, which was much lower than the agreed-upon 15 minutes per session. Ms. Blake noticed that Xander was coming to her room late for this intervention period. Xander had been going to other teachers to receive help with homework first before coming to the math room during her study skills block. Mr. Wilson and Ms. Blake talked to Xander and his study skills teacher to problem-solve this situation. Together they agreed that Xander would come to the math room first during her study skills block and seek extra help in other subjects if he had time. If this did not provide enough time for Xander to get the subject-area help he needed, Xander, the teachers, and his parents agreed that he could access that help in the after-school homework program. Mr. Wilson documented this update on the implementation plan.

After the meeting, Mr. Wilson completed the Fidelity Data Sheet for Self-Monitoring (Appendix 8.2), documented the provision of this support on the Implementation Tracking Log (see Figure 11.25), finalized the self-monitoring form and provided copies to Ms. Blake, and checked in with her after a week of self-monitoring to see how it was going and to answer any questions.

MS. MORALES: PERFORMANCE-BUILDING IMPLEMENTATION SUPPORT— REVISE THE IMPLEMENTATION PLAN

Before deciding to provide a new implementation support, Mr. Wilson checked in with Ms. Morales to discuss any barriers she was experiencing to consistently providing students with rewards. Ms. Morales indicated that it was easy to provide students with tangible rewards (e.g., candy, notebooks, homework passes), but more difficult to arrange the activity-based rewards, especially when they involved preferred adults (e.g., basketball game, special lunch). Currently, when a student reached his or her goal and chose an activity-based reward, Ms. Morales would email the preferred adult to inform him or her of the specific reward activity and to schedule one. Mr. Wilson suggested that as soon as a student chose an activity with a preferred adult as a possible reward, Ms. Morales (1) inform the adult of the student who had selected him or her and the activity chosen, (2) confirm that the adult is willing to be part of the reward plan, (3) identify times and days that are generally feasible for the adult to engage in the activity, and (4) inform the adult to plan ahead because the student had only one more day to meet his or her goal before earning a reward. Mr. Wilson created a CICO reward calendar that was shared with the relevant staff to help everyone stay organized and accountable. This modification was documented in the implementation plan, and after the meeting, Mr. Wilson documented the provision of this support on the Implementation Tracking Log (see Figure 11.25).

MR. RODRIGUEZ: SKILL-BUILDING IMPLEMENTATION SUPPORT—ROLE PLAY

Mr. Rodriguez inconsistently completed the CICO form across students and did not prompt behavioral expectations at the beginning of class. Mr. Wilson decided to implement role play as a skill-building implementation support to specifically target these intervention steps and provide additional practice to promote fluency with implementing the entire intervention. Before meeting with Mr. Rodriguez, Mr. Wilson reviewed the intervention rationale and available data (learner outcomes for Mr. Rodriguez's specific class period and intervention fidelity). He confirmed the steps he wanted to practice with Mr. Rodriguez and decided on an order for role-playing these steps that mirrored what happened in the typical classroom setting. He gathered the needed materials and arranged to meet with Mr. Rodriguez. At the meeting, Mr. Wilson first explained the purpose of role playing and what it entailed (i.e., identifying challenging implementation scenarios; role playing a scenario, with Mr. Wilson as the implementer and Mr. Rodriguez as the student; switching roles for a new scenario). Mr. Rodriguez identified a goal for the implementation session: Develop fluency in providing feedback to students at the end of the class while completing the CICO form (Step 1). Mr. Wilson described the importance of the intervention in relation to supporting the students' consistent demonstration of schoolwide behavioral expectations and how implementation of CICO impacts learner outcomes (Step 2). He further explained the relation between high levels of intervention fidelity over time and improvements in learner outcomes. Mr. Wilson reviewed intervention fidelity graphs, highlighting the areas in which Mr. Rodriguez was consistently performing (e.g., providing praise) and the areas requiring additional practice (e.g., prompting behavioral expectations, completing the CICO form, and providing feedback) because they were implemented inconsistently (Step 3). Mr. Rodriguez agreed that these were the steps he wanted to practice during role play (Step 4). He thought that practicing the prompting of behavioral expectations as soon as students were transitioned into the classroom, and rating student behavior and providing CICO ratings and feedback when students were completing work at the end of the class period would be good practice scenarios (Step 5). Mr. Wilson demonstrated prompting behavioral expectations (Step 6). He noted that, at the beginning of class, he could (1) remind the student privately of one important behavioral expectation to follow (e.g., "You did a great job with staying in your seat yesterday. Today let's focus on keeping conversations directed toward the story we're reading—I think you're really going to like this one!") or (2) provide the whole class with a prompt for following behavioral expectations (e.g., "Let's all remember to let classmates who have been called on finish sharing their ideas before someone else has a turn to talk; I will call on students who have their hands raised and are sitting quietly"). The latter might be more feasible at the beginning of class, but either way, Mr. Rodriguez should offer encouragement and specific praise for following behavioral expectations to the target student throughout the class period. After Mr. Wilson demonstrated different ways to prompt behavioral expectations at the beginning of class, he showed Mr. Rodriguez how to provide CICO ratings and feedback, and then discussed the demonstration with Mr. Rodriguez (Step 7). Then Mr. Rodriguez practiced. They reviewed the step he was going to practice (i.e., providing CICO ratings and feedback). Mr. Rodriguez determined that he wanted to focus on providing feedback in a praise–correct–praise format. Mr. Rodriguez then role-played providing feedback when the student had earned all but one of his or her points (Step 8). Mr. Wilson suggested that they also practice when a student has a more challenging day behaviorally and may receive ratings of 1 and 0. Mr. Rodriguez focused on remaining neutral and encouraging what the student could do in the next class to improve his or her ratings. Mr. Wilson also let Mr. Rodriguez know that if a student earned ratings of 2 throughout the class, there was no need to try to find something to correct; he could just offer praise and encouragement. At the end of practice, Mr. Rodriguez said he felt much more confident about providing feedback. Before this intervention with Mr. Wilson, Mr. Rodriguez had thought that the feedback needed to take longer, which is why he didn't always provide ratings or provide feedback—he would run out of time at the end of class. Mr. Wilson reinforced the point that the feedback only needs to take a minute or 2, and if Mr. Rodriguez needed to start providing feedback a few minutes earlier in the class period, he could do so (Step 9). Mr. Wilson ended the meeting by reviewing what they had accomplished and thanking Mr. Rodriguez for practicing the different intervention steps (Step 10). After the meeting, Mr. Wilson completed the Fidelity Data Sheet for Role Play (Appendix 7.4) and documented the provision of the role play support on the Implementation Tracking Log (see Figure 11.25). A few days later, he checked in with Mr. Rodriguez to answer any questions.

Step 11: Evaluate the Intervention

After the provision of varied implementation supports, all implementers were providing the CICO intervention with high levels of adherence (i.e., over 90%; see Figure 11.39). This level of implementation would likely support improved learner outcomes. Further,

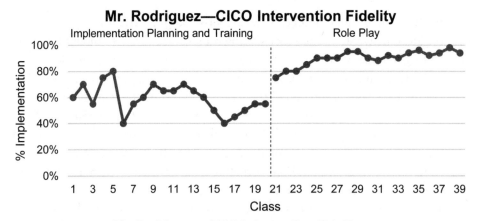

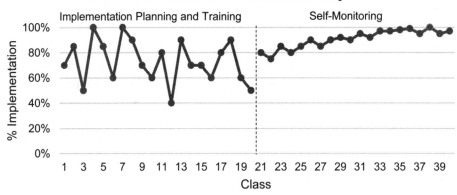

(continued)

FIGURE 11.39. Intervention fidelity data after implementation supports.

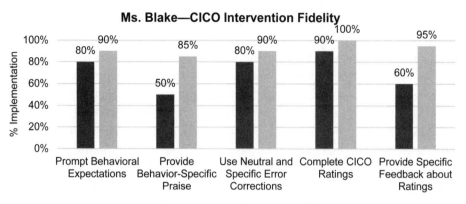

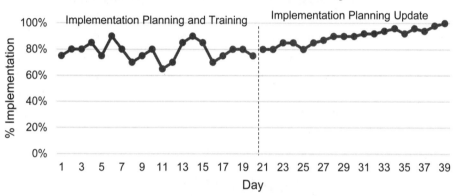

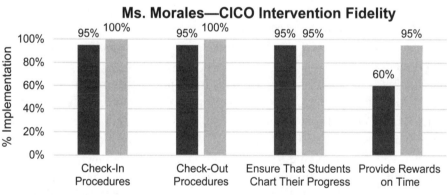

FIGURE 11.39. *(continued)*

Xander received the appropriate dosage (i.e., 15 minutes daily) of the math accuracy intervention on 95% of days.

After 2 months of implementation, both Anthony and Gloria met their CICO point goal and were working toward maintaining this behavioral improvement (see Figure 11.40). Given sufficient intervention fidelity and greatly improved learner outcomes, Anthony and Gloria's data now fit within Data Profile A. The intervention will be continued as written and learner outcome and intervention fidelity data will continue to be reviewed regularly.

Xander was experiencing mixed outcomes with the interventions he was receiving (see Figure 11.40). After Xander received the math accuracy intervention for the correct amount of time (i.e., 15 minutes daily instead of 5 minutes), his rate of progress increased steadily. He did not meet his goal of 80% of problems correct in a 2-month period, but the team decided to continue with the current intervention, given his recent improvements and adequate implementation. Xander's response to sufficient intervention fidelity of the CICO intervention was not as robust. He only increased her percentage of points earned to 75%, instead of his goal of 85%. The team noticed that Xander went long stretches without earning a reward. To increase his motivation, they changed the criteria to earn a reward from 4 nonconsecutive days of meeting the target percentage to 2 nonconsecutive days. They decided to try this format for 2 weeks, review the data, and then determine if an alternative intervention should be implemented. Evaluating the intervention was documented on the Implementation Tracking Log (see Figure 11.25).

CONCLUSION

These case studies illustrate the processes and strategies described in this book put into action to support implementers and improve learner outcomes. By collecting and evaluating intervention fidelity, the consultants in these cases were able to ensure that the research-based interventions were delivered as planned. In doing so, they maximized learner outcomes. In practice, intervention fidelity assessment and implementation support strategies are rarely used in school settings, despite their necessity. As a result, learner outcomes have been poorer than they could be. By using the processes and strategies in this book, you can support implementers by applying research- and data-based implementation strategies to improve intervention fidelity and subsequently learner outcomes. Until implementation is consistently and comprehensively addressed, we are never going to realize the benefits of evidence-based practice; we will make little to no meaningful progress for learners in need of intervention.

By using the model and strategies in this book, you will be (1) at the forefront of implementation, (2) responsive to implementers who need support, (3) upholding your ethical and legal obligations, (4) giving learners in need of intervention an opportunity to make meaningful progress, and (5) working efficiently. We hope you will use this model as a framework to individualize the intervention fidelity data collection, decisions, and supports appropriate to the learners and implementers in your context.

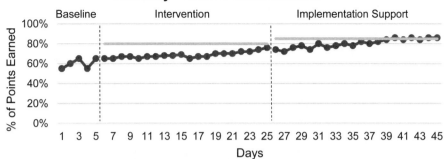

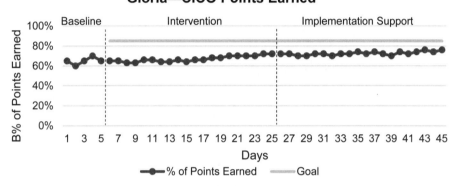

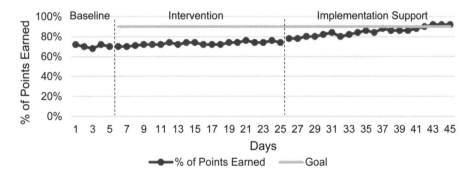

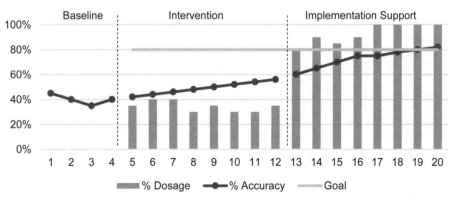

FIGURE 11.40. Learner data after intervention and implementation support.

References

Algozzine, B., Barrett, S., Eber, L., George, H., Horner, R., Lewis, T., . . . Sugai, G (2014). School-wide PBIS Tiered Fidelity Inventory. Retrieved from *www.pbis.org*.

Allinder, R. M., Bolling, R. M., Oats, R. G., & Gagnon, W. A. (2000). Effects of teacher self-monitoring on implementation of curriculum-based measurement and mathematics computation achievement of students with disabilities. *Remedial and Special Education, 21,* 219–226.

Altschaefl, M., & Kratochwill, T. R. (2016). *Promoting treatment integrity of parent- and teacher-delivered math fluency interventions: An adult behavior change intervention.* Manuscript in preparation.

American Counseling Association. (2014). *Code of ethics.* Alexandria, VA: Author.

Ammentorp, J., Kofoed, P., & Laulund, L. W. (2010). Impact of communication skills training on parents' perceptions of care: Intervention study. *Journal of Advanced Nursing, 67*(2), 394–400.

Baker, R. C., & Kirschenbaum, D. S. (1993). Self-monitoring may be necessary for successful weight control. *Behavior Therapy, 24,* 377–394.

Bandura, A. (1977). *Social learning theory.* New York: General Learning Press.

Barrish, H. H., Saunders, M., & Wolf, M. M. (1969). Good behavior game: Effects of individual contingencies for group consequences on disruptive behavior in a classroom. *Journal of Applied Behavior Analysis, 2,* 119–124.

Behavior Analyst Certification Board. (2014). *Professional and ethical compliance code.* Littleton, CO: Author.

Belfiore, P. J., Fritts, K. M., & Herman, B. C. (2008). The role of procedural integrity: Using self-monitoring to enhance discrete trial instruction. *Focus on Autism and Other Developmental Disabilities, 23,* 95–102.

Bergan, J. R., & Kratochwill, T. R. (1990). *Behavioral consultation in applied settings.* New York: Plenum Press.

Bice-Urbach, B., & Kratochwill, T. R. (2016). Teleconsultation: The use of technology to improve evidence-based practices in rural communities. *Journal of School Psychology, 56,* 27–43.

Braswell, L., & Kendall, P. C. (2001). Cognitive-behavioral therapy with youth. In K. S. Dobson (Ed.), *Handbook of cognitive-behavioral therapies* (2nd ed., pp. 246–294). New York: Guilford Press.

Briesch, A. M., & Chafouleas, S. M. (2009). Review and analysis of literature on self-management interventions to promote appropriate classroom behaviors (1988–2008). *School Psychology Quarterly, 24,* 106–118.

Burke, R. V., Howard, M. R., Peterson, J. L., Peterson, R. W., & Allen, K. D. (2012). Visual performance feedback: Effects on targeted and nontargeted staff. *Behavior Modification, 36*(5), 687–704.

Byron, J. R., & Sanetti, L. M. H. (2018). *Implementation planning as a proactive approach to treatment integrity maintenance of an academic intervention.* Manuscript under review.

Chafouleas, S. M., Riley-Tillman, T. C., & Sugai, G. (2007). *School-based behavioral assessment: Informing instruction and intervention.* New York: Guilford Press.

Chorpita, B. F. (2007). *Modular cognitive-behavioral therapy for childhood anxiety disorders.* New York: Guilford Press.

Codding, R. S., & Lane, K. L. (2015). A spotlight on treatment intensity: An important and often overlooked component of intervention inquiry. *Journal of Behavioral Education, 24,* 1–10.

Codding, R. S., Livanis, A., Pace, G. M., & Vaca, L. (2008). Using performance to improve implementation of a class-wide behavior support plan: Examining observer reactivity. *Journal of Applied Behavior Analysis, 41,* 417–422.

Codding, R., Sanetti, L. M. H., & DiGennaro Reed, F. M. (2014). Best practices in facilitating consultation and collaboration with teachers and administrators. In P. Harrison & A. Thomas (Eds.), *Best practices in school psychology: Data-based and collaborative decision making* (6th ed., pp. 525–540). Bethesda, MD: National Association of School Psychologists.

Collier-Meek, M. A., Fallon, L. M., & DeFouw, E. R. (2017). Towards feasible implementation support: Emailed prompts to promote teachers' treatment integrity. *School Psychology Review, 46,* 379–394.

Collier-Meek, M. A., Fallon, L. M., & DeFouw, E. R. (2018). Assessing implementation of the Good Behavior Game: Comparing estimates of adherence, quality, and exposure. *Assessment for Effective Intervention.* [Epub ahead of print]

Collier-Meek, M. A., Fallon, L. M., & Gould, K. (2018). How are treatment integrity data assessed?: Reviewing the performance feedback literature. *School Psychology Quarterly.* [Epub ahead of print]

Collier-Meek, M. A., Fallon, L. M., Sanetti, L. M. H., & Maggin, D. M. (2013). Focus on implementation: Assessing and promoting treatment fidelity. *TEACHING Exceptional Children, 45,* 52–59.

Collier-Meek, M. A., Johnson, A. H., & Farrell, A. F. (2018). Development and initial evaluation of the Measure of Active Supervision and Interaction in out-of-school time. *Assessment for Effective Intervention, 43,* 212–226.

Collier-Meek, M. A., Sanetti, L. M. H., & Boyle, A. M. (2016). Providing feasible implementation support: Direct training and implementation planning in consultation. *School Psychology Forum, 10,* 106–119.

Collier-Meek, M. A., Sanetti, L. M. H., Levin, J., Kratochwill, T. R., & Boyle, A. M. (2018). *Evaluating the impact implementation supports on teachers' classroom management and class-wide behavior.* Manuscript submitted for publication.

Cooper, J. O., Heron, T. E., & Heward, W. L. (2007). *Applied behavior analysis* (2nd ed.). Upper Saddle River, NJ: Pearson.

Council for Exceptional Children. (2015). *Ethical principles and professional practice standards for special educators.* Arlington, VA: Author.

Dart, E. H., Cook, C. R., Collins, T. A., Gresham, F. M., & Chenier, J. S. (2012). Test driving interventions to increase treatment integrity and student outcomes. *School Psychology Review, 41,* 467–481.

Dib, N., & Sturmey, P. (2007). Reducing student stereotypy by improving teachers' implementation of discrete-trial teaching. *Journal of Applied Behavior Analysis, 40,* 339–343.

DiGennaro Reed, F. D., & Codding, R. S. (2014). Advancements in procedural fidelity assessment and intervention: Introduction to the special issue. *Journal of Behavioral Education, 23,* 1–18.

DiGennaro Reed, F. D., Codding, R. S., Catania, C. N., & Maguire, H. (2010). Effects of video modeling on treatment integrity of behavioral interventions. *Journal of Applied Behavior Analysis, 43,* 291–295.

DiGennaro Reed, F. D., Reed, D. D., Baez, C. N., & Maguire, H. (2011). A parametric analysis of errors of commission during discrete-trial training. *Journal of Applied Behavior Analysis, 44,* 611–615.

Dobson, K. S. (Ed.). (2010). *Handbook of cognitive-behavioral therapies* (3rd ed.). New York: Guilford Press.

Downs, A. F., Rosenthal, T. L., & Lichstein, K. L. (1988). Modeling therapies reduces avoidance of bath-time by the institutionalized elderly. *Behavior Therapy, 19*(3), 359–368.

Draxten, M., Flattum, C., & Fulkerson, J. (2016). An example of how to supplement goal setting to promote behavior change for families using motivational interviewing. *Health Communication, 31,* 1276–1283.

Dufrene, B. A., Parker, K., Menousek, K., Zhou, Q., Harpole, L., & Olmi, D. J. (2012). Direct behavioral consultation in Head Start to increase teacher use of praise and effective instruction delivery. *Journal of Educational and Psychological Consultation, 22,* 159–186.

Duhon, G. J., Noell, G. H., Witt, J. C., & Freeland, J. T. (2004). Identifying academic skill and performance deficits: The experimental analysis of brief assessments of academic skills. *School Psychology Review, 33,* 429–443.

Durlak, J. A., & DuPre, E. P. (2008). Implementation matters: A review of research on the influence of implementation on program outcomes and the factors affecting implementation. *American Journal of Community Psychology, 41,* 327–350.

Eames, C., Daley D., Hutchings, J., Hughes, J. C., Jones, K., Martin, P., & Bywater, T. (2007) The Leader Observation Tool: A process skills treatment fidelity measure for the Incredible Years parenting programme. *Child: Care, Health and Development, 34,* 391–400.

Ennett, S. T., Ringwalt, C. L., Thorne, J., Rohrbach, L. A., Vincus, A., Simons-Rudolph, A., & Jones, S. (2003). A comparison of current practice in school-based substance use prevention programs within meta-analysis findings. *Prevention Science, 4,* 1–14.

Every Student Succeeds Act. (2015). Public Law No. 114-95 § 114 Stat. 1177.

Fallon, L. M., Collier-Meek, M. A., Maggin, D. M., Sanetti, L. M. H., & Johnson, A. H. (2015). Is performance feedback an evidence-based intervention?: A systematic review and evaluation of single-case research. *Exceptional Children, 8,* 227–246.

Fallon, L. M., Collier-Meek, M. A., Sanetti, L. M. H., Feinberg, A., & Kratochwill, T. R. (2016). Implementation planning to promote parents' treatment integrity of behavioral interventions for children with autism. *Journal of Educational and Psychological Consultation, 26,* 87–109.

Fallon, L. M., Kurtz, K. D., & Mueller, M. R. (2018). Direct training to improve educators' treatment integrity: A systematic review of single-case design studies. *School Psychology Quarterly, 33*(2), 169–181.

Fallon, L. M., Sanetti, L. M. H., Chafouleas, S. M., Faggella-Luby, M. N., & Welch, M. E. (2018). Direct training to increase agreement of treatment integrity ratings. *Assessment for Effective Intervention, 43,* 196–211.

Fantuzzo, J. W., & Polite, K. (1990). School-based, behavioral self-management: A review and analysis. *School Psychology Quarterly, 5,* 180–198.

Fischer, A. J., Schultz, B. K., Collier-Meek, M. A., Zoder-Martell, K., & Erchul, W. P. (2018). A critical review of videoconferencing software to support school consultation. *International Journal of School and Educational Psychology, 6,* 12–22.

Fixsen, D. L., Blasé, K. A., Duda, M. A., Naoom, S. F., & Van Dyke, M. (2010). Implementation of evidence-based treatments for children and adolescents: Research findings and their implications for the future. In J. R. Weisz & A. E. Kazdin (Eds.), *Evidence-based psychotherapies for children and adolescents* (pp. 435–450). New York: Guilford Press.

Fixsen, D. L., Naoom, S. F., Blasé, K. A., Friedman, R. M., & Wallace, F. (2005). *Implementation research: A synthesis of the literature.* Tampa, FL: University of South Florida, Louis de la Parte Florida Mental Health Institute, The National Implementation Research Network (FMHI Publication No. 231). Retrieved November 1, 2015, from *http://nirn.fmhi.usf.edu/resources/publications/Monograph/pdf/monograph_full.pdf.*

Forman, S. G., Shapiro, E. S., Codding, R. S., Gonzales, J. E., Reddy, L. A., Rosenfield, S. A., . . . Stoiber, K. C. (2013). Implementation science and school psychology. *School Psychology Quarterly, 28,* 77–100.

Frey, A. J., Sims, K., & Alvarez, M. E. (2013). The promise of motivational interviewing for securing a niche in the RtI movement. *Children and Schools, 35,* 67–70.

Frey, J. R., Elliott, S. N., & Miller, C. F. (2014). Best practices in social skills training. In. P. L. Harrison & A. Thomas (Eds.), *Best practices in school psychology: Student-level services* (pp. 231–224). Bethesda, MD: National Association of School Psychologists.

Fuchs, D., & Fuchs, L. S. (2017). Critique of the national evaluation of response to intervention: A case for simpler frameworks. *Exceptional Children, 83,* 255–268.

Gilbertson, D., Witt, J. C., Singletary, L. L., & VanDerHeyden, A. (2007). Supporting teacher use of interventions: Effects of response dependent performance feedback on teacher implementation of a math intervention. *Journal of Behavioral Education, 16,* 311–326.

Gresham, F. M. (2014). Measuring and analyzing treatment integrity in research. In L. Sanetti & T. Kratochwill (Eds.), *Treatment integrity: A foundation for evidence-based practice in applied psychology* (pp. 109–130). Washington, DC: American Psychological Association.

Hettema, J., Ernst, D., Williams, J. R., & Miller, K. J. (2014). Parallel processes: Using motivational interviewing as an implementation coaching strategy. *Journal of Behavioral Health Services and Research, 41,* 324–336.

Hettema, J., Steele, J., & Miller, W. R. (2005). Motivational interviewing. *Annual Review of Clinical Psychology, 1,* 91–111.

Hirschstein, M. K., Edstrom, L. V., Frey, K. S., Snell, J. L., & MacKenzie, E. P. (2007). Walking the talk in bully prevention: Teacher implementation variables related to initial impact of the Steps to Respect program. *School Psychology Review, 36,* 3–21.

Hood, C., & Dorman, D. (2008). Best practices in the display of data. In A. Thomas & J. Grimes (Eds.), *Best practices in school psychology V* (Vol. 6, pp. 2117–2132). Bethseda, MD: National Association of School Psychologists.

Horner, R. H., Carr, E. G., Halle, J., McGee, G., Odom, S., & Wolery, M. (2005). The use of single-subject research to identify evidence-based practice in special education. *Exceptional Children, 71,* 165–179.

Individuals with Disabilities Education Act. (2004). 20 U.S.C. § 1400.

Jeffrey, J. L., McCurdy, B. L., Ewing, S., & Polis, D. (2009). Classwide PBIS for students with EBD: Initial evaluation of an integrity tool. *Education and Treatment of Children, 32,* 537–550.

Jenkins, S. R., & DiGennaro Reed, F. D. (2016). A parametric analysis of rehearsal opportunities on procedural integrity. *Journal of Organizational Behavior Management, 36,* 255–281.

Joyce, B., & Showers, B. (2002). *Student achievement through staff development* (3rd ed.). Alexandria, VA: Association for Supervision and Curriculum Development.

Kazdin, A. E. (2013). *Behavior modification in applied settings.* Long Grove, IL: Waveland Press.

Kazdin, A. E., & Weisz, J. R. (2010). Introduction: Context, background, and goals. In A. E. Kazdin

& J. R. Weisz (Eds.), *Evidence-based psychotherapies for children and adolescents* (pp. 3–9). New York: Guilford Press.

Kilgus, S. P., Collier-Meek, M. A., Johnson, A. H., & Jaffery, R. (2014). Applied empiricism: Ensuring the validity of response-to-intervention decisions. *Contemporary School Psychology, 18*, 1–12.

Kitsantas, A. (2000). The role of self-regulation strategies and self-efficacy perceptions in successful weight loss maintenance. *Psychology and Health, 15*, 811–820.

Knight, J., Elford, M., Hock, M., Dunekack, D., Bradley, B., Deshler, D. D., & Knight, D. (2015). 3 steps to great coaching: A simple but powerful instructional coaching cycle nets results. *Journal of Staff Development, 36*, 11–18.

Kratochwill, T. R., Altschaefl, M. R., & Bice-Urbach, B. (2014). Best practices in school-based problem-solving consultation: Applications in prevention and intervention systems. In A. Thomas & P. L. Harrison (Eds.), *Best practices in school psychology VI: Data-based and collaborative decision making* (pp. 461–482). Bethesda, MD: National Association of School Psychologists.

Kratochwill, T. R., & Bergan, J. R. (1990). *Behavioral consultation in applied settings: An individual guide.* New York: Plenum Press.

Kratochwill, T. R., Hitchcock, J., Horner, R. H., Levin, J. R., Odom, S. L., Rindskopf, D. M., & Shadish, W. R. (2010). Single-case designs technical documentation. Retrieved from *http://ies.ed.gov/ncee/wwc/pdf/wwc_scd.pdf.*

Long, A. C. J., Sanetti, L. M. H., Lark, C. R., & Connolly, J. G. (2018). Examining behavioral consultation plus computer-based implementation planning on teachers' intervention implementation in an alternative school. *Remedial and Special Education, 39*, 106–117.

Lylo, B. J., & Lee, D. L. (2013). Effects of delayed audio-based self-monitoring on teacher completion of learning trials. *Journal of Behavioral Education, 22*, 120–138.

McHugh, R. K., & Barlow, D. H. (2010). The dissemination and implementation of evidence-based treatments. *American Psychologist, 65*, 73–84.

Miles, N. I., & Wilder, D. A. (2009). The effects of behavioral skills training on caregiver implementation of guided compliance. *Journal of Applied Behavior Analysis, 42*, 405–410.

Miller, W. R., & Rollnick, S. (2013). *Motivational interviewing: Helping people change* (3rd ed.). New York: Guilford Press.

Minor, S. W., Minor, J. W., & Williams, P. P. (1983). A participant modeling procedure to train parents of developmentally disabled infants. *Journal of Psychology: Interdisciplinary and Applied, 115*, 107–111.

Mouzakitis, A., Codding, R. S., & Tryon, G. (2015). The effects of self-monitoring and performance feedback on the treatment integrity of behavior intervention plan implementation and generalization. *Journal of Positive Behavior Interventions, 17*, 223–234.

National Association of School Psychologists. (2010). *Principles for professional ethics.* Bethesda, MD: Author.

National Center on Response to Intervention. (2010). Essential components of RTI: A closer look at response to intervention. Retrieved from *www.rti4success.org.*

Newman, E. J., & Tuckman, B. W. (1997). The effects of participant modeling on self-efficacy, incentive, productivity, and performance. *Journal of Research and Development in Education, 31*(1), 38–45.

Nilsen, P. (2015). Making sense of implementation theories, models and frameworks. *Implementation Science, 10*, 53.

Noell, G. H., & Gansle, K. A. (2006). Assuring the form has substance: Treatment plan implementation as the foundation of assessing response to intervention. *Assessment for Effective Intervention, 32*, 32–39.

Noell, G. H., & Gansle, K. A. (2013). The use of performance feedback to improve intervention implementation in schools. In L. M. H. Sanetti & T. R. Kratochwill (Eds.), *Treatment integrity: A foundation for evidence-based practice in applied psychology* (pp. 161–184). Washington, DC: American Psychological Association.

Noell, G. H., Gansle, K. A., Meyers, J. L., Knox, R. M., Mintz, J. C., & Danhir, A. (2014). Improving treatment plan implementation in schools: A meta-analysis of single-subject design studies. *Journal of Behavioral Education, 23,* 168–191.

Noell, G. H., Witt, J. C., Gilbertson, D. N., Ranier, D. D., & Freeland, J. T. (1997). Increasing teacher intervention implementation in general education settings through consultation and performance feedback. *School Psychology Quarterly, 12,* 77–88.

Noell, G. H., Witt, J. C., Slider, N. J., Connell, J. E., Gatti, S. L., Williams, K. L., . . . Duhon, D. J. (2005). Treatment implementation following behavioral consultation in schools: A comparison of three follow-up strategies. *School Psychology Review, 34,* 87–106.

O'Halloran, P. D., Shields, N., Blackstock, F., Wintle, E., & Taylor, N. F. (2016). Motivational interviewing increases physical activity and self-efficacy in people living in the community after hip fracture: A randomized controlled trial. *Clinical Rehabilitation, 30,* 1108–1119.

Ollendick, T. H., & King, N. J. (1998). Empirically supported treatments for children with phobic and anxiety disorders: Current status. *Journal of Clinical Child Psychology, 27*(2), 156–167.

Perepletchikova, F., & Kazdin, A. E. (2005). Treatment integrity and therapeutic change: Issues and research recommendations. *Clinical Psychology: Science and Practice, 12,* 365–383.

Petscher, E. S., & Bailey, J. S. (2006). Effects of training, prompting, and self-monitoring on staff behavior in a classroom for students with disabilities. *Journal of Applied Behavior Analysis, 39,* 215–226.

Plavnick, J. B., Ferreri, S. J., & Maupin, A. N. (2010). The effects of self-monitoring on the procedural integrity of a behavioral intervention for young children with developmental disabilities. *Journal of Applied Behavior Analysis, 43,* 315–320.

Power, T. J., Blom-Hoffman, J., Clarke, A. T., Riley-Tillman, T. C., Kellerher, C., & Manz, P. (2005). Reconceptualizing intervention integrity: A partnership-based framework for linking research with practice. *Psychology in the Schools, 42,* 495–507.

Ransford, C. R., Greenberg, M. T., Domitrovich, C. E., Small, M., & Jacobson, L. (2009). The role of teachers' psychological experiences and perceptions of curriculum supports on the implementation of a social and emotional learning curriculum. *School Psychology Review, 38,* 510–532.

Reddy, L. A., Fabiano, G., Dudek, C. M., & Hsu, L. (2013). Development and construct validity of the Classroom Strategies Scale—Observer Form. *School Psychology Quarterly, 28,* 317–341.

Reinke, W. M., Lewis-Palmer, T., & Merrell, K. (2008). The classroom check-up: A classwide teacher consultation model for increasing praise and decreasing disruptive behavior. *School Psychology Review, 37,* 315–332.

Riley-Tillman, T. C., & Burns, M. K. (2009). *Evaluating educational interventions: Single-case design for measuring response to intervention.* New York: Guilford Press.

Ringwalt, C. L., Ennett, S., Johnson, R., Rohrbach, L. A., Simons-Rudolph, A., Vincus, A., & Thorne, J. (2003). Factors associated with fidelity to substance use prevention curriculum guides in the nation's middle schools. *Health Education and Behavior, 30,* 375–391.

Romi, S., & Teichman, M. (1998). Participant modelling training programme: Tutoring the paraprofessional. *British Journal of Guidance and Counselling, 26*(2), 297–301.

Rosenfield, S. A. (1987). *Instructional consultation.* Hillsdale, NJ: Erlbaum.

Sanetti, L. M. H., & Collier-Meek, M. A. (2014). Increasing the rigor of treatment integrity assessment: A comparison of direct observation and permanent product methods. *Journal of Behavioral Education 23,* 60–88.

Sanetti, L. M. H., & Collier-Meek, S. M. (2015). Data-driven delivery of implementation supports in a multi-tiered framework: A pilot study. *Psychology in the Schools, 52*, 815–828.

Sanetti, L. M. H., Collier-Meek, M. A., Long, A. C. J., Byron, J. R., & Kratochwill, T. R. (2015). Increasing teacher treatment integrity of behavior support plans through consultation and implementation planning. *Journal of School Psychology, 53*, 209–229.

Sanetti, L. M. H., Collier-Meek, M. A., Long, A. C. J., Kim, J., & Kratochwill, T. R. (2014). Using implementation planning to increase teachers' adherence and quality to behavior support plans. *Psychology in the Schools, 51*, 879–895.

Sanetti, L. M. H., & Fallon, L. M. (2011). Treatment integrity assessment: How estimates of adherence, quality, and exposure influence interpretation of implementation. *Journal of Educational and Psychological Consultation, 21*, 209–232.

Sanetti, L. M. H., Fallon, L. M., Collier-Meek, M. A. (2011). Treatment integrity assessment and intervention by school-based personnel: Practical applications based on a preliminary study. *School Psychology Forum, 5*(3), 87–102.

Sanetti, L. M. H., & Kratochwill, T. R. (2009). Toward developing a science of treatment integrity: Introduction to the special series. *School Psychology Review, 38*, 445–459. Retrieved from *www.nasponline.org/publications/spr/spr384index.aspx.*

Sanetti, L. M. H., Kratochwill, T. R., & Long, A. C. J. (2013). Applying adult behavior change theory to support mediator-based intervention implementation. *School Psychology Quarterly, 28*, 47–62.

Sanetti, L. M. H., Luiselli, J., & Handler, M. (2007). Effects of verbal and graphic performance feedback on behavior support plan implementation in an inclusion classroom. *Behavior Modification, 31*, 454–465.

Sanetti, L. M. H., Williamson, K. M., Long, A. C. J., & Kratochwill, T. R. (2018). Increasing inservice teacher implementation of classroom management practices through consultation, implementation planning, and participant modeling. *Journal of Positive Behavior Interventions, 20*(1), 43–59.

Sarokoff, R. A., & Sturmey, P. (2004). The effects of behavioral skills training on staff implementation of discrete-trial teaching. *Journal of Applied Behavior Analysis, 37*, 535–538.

Scholz, U., Schüz, B., Ziegelmann, J. P., Lippke, S., & Schwarzer, R. (2008). Beyond behavioural intentions: Planning mediates between intentions and physical activity. *British Journal of Health Psychology, 13*, 479–494.

Schulte, A. C., Easton, J. E., & Parker, J. (2009). Advances in treatment integrity research: Multidisciplinary perspectives on the conceptualization, measurement, and enhancement of treatment integrity. *School Psychology Review, 38*, 460–475.

Schultz, B. K., Arora, P., & Mautone, J. A. (2015). Consultants and coaching to increase the uptake of evidence-based practices: Introduction to the special issue. *School Mental Health, 7*, 1–5.

Schwarzer, R. (1992). Self-efficacy in the adoption and maintenance of health behaviors: Theoretical approaches and a new model. In R. Schwarzer (Ed.), *Self-efficacy: Thought control of action* (pp. 217–243). Washington, DC: Hemisphere.

Schwarzer, R. (2008). Modeling health behavior change: How to predict and modify the adoption and maintenance of health behaviors. *Applied Psychology: An International Review, 57*, 1–29.

Sheridan, S. M., & Kratochwill, T. R. (2007). *Conjoint behavioral consultation: Promoting family–school connections and interventions.* New York: Springer.

Simonsen, B., MacSuga, A. S., Fallon, L. M., & Sugai, G. (2013). The effects of self-monitoring on teachers' use of specific praise. *Journal of Positive Behavior Interventions, 15*, 5–15.

Skinner, C. H., McLaughlin, T. F., & Logan, P. (1997). Cover, copy, and compare: A self-managed academic intervention effective across skills, students, and settings. *Journal of Behavioral Education, 7*, 295–306.

Sniehotta, F. F., Scholz, U., & Schwarzer, R. (2005). Bridging the intention–behavior gap: Planning, self-efficacy, and action control in the adoption and maintenance of physical exercise. *Psychology and Health, 20*, 143–160.

Solomon, B. G., Klein, S. A., & Politylo, B. C. (2012). The effect of performance feedback on teachers' treatment integrity: A meta-analysis of the single-case literature. *School Psychology Review, 41*, 160–175.

Sterling-Turner, H. E., Watson, T. S., & Moore, J. W. (2002). The effects of direct training and treatment integrity on treatment outcomes in school consultation. *School Psychology Quarterly, 17*, 47–77.

Sterling-Turner, H., Watson, T. S., Wildmon, M., Watkins, C., & Little, E. (2001). Investigating the relationship between training type and treatment integrity. *School Psychology Quarterly, 16*, 56–67.

Stoiber, K. C., & DeSmet, J. (2010). Guildelines for evidence-based practice in selecting interventions. In R. Ervin, G. Peacock, E. Daly, & K. Merrell (Eds.), *Practical handbook of school psychology* (pp. 213–234). New York: Guilford Press.

Sundman-Wheat, A. N., Bradley-Klug, K. L., & Ogg, J. A. (2012). Investigation of a parent-directed intervention designed to promote early literacy skills in preschool children. *Journal of Evidence-Based Practices for Schools, 13*, 172–199.

Thompson, M. T., Marchant, M., Anderson, D., Prater, M. A., & Gibb, G. (2012). Effects of tiered training on general educators' use of specific praise. *Education and Treatment of Children, 35*, 521–546.

Trijsburg, R. W., Jelicic, M., van den Broek, W. W., & Plekker, A. E. M. (1996). Exposure and participant modelling in a case of injection phobia. *Psychotherapy and Psychosomatics, 65*(1), 57–61.

Walker, D. D., Walton, T. O., Neighbors, C., Kaysen, D., Mbilinyi, L., Darnell, J., . . . Roffman, R. A. (2017). Randomized trial of motivational interviewing plus feedback for soldiers with untreated alcohol abuse. *Journal of Consulting and Clinical Psychology, 85*, 99–110.

Wilder, D. A., Atwell, J., & Wine, B. (2006). The effects of varying levels of treatment integrity on child compliance during treatment with a three-step prompting procedure. *Journal of Applied Behavior Analysis, 39*, 369–373.

Winett, R. A., Kramer, K. D., Walker, W. B., Malone, S. W., & Lane, M. K. (1988). Modifying food purchases in supermarkets with modeling, feedback, and goal-setting procedures. *Journal of Applied Behavior Analysis, 21*(1), 73–80.

Wright, J. (2013). How to: Deliver direct instruction in general-education classrooms. Retrieved from *www.interventioncentral.org/sites/default/files/pdfs/pdfs_blog/instruction_direct_instruction.pdf.*

Yamamoto, S., Kagami, Y., Ogura, M., & Isawa, S. (2013). Effects of basic social skills training and simulation training on acquisition of social skills related to employment: Adults with high-functioning pervasive developmental disorders. *Japanese Journal of Special Education, 51*(3), 291–299.

Index

Note. *f* or *t* following a page number indicates a figure or a table.